As Executive Director of the King County Medical Society, I have come to know Doctor Johnson over these past fifteen years as a warm-hearted, genuine, and caring physician to his patients. Doctor Paul, as we know him in Seattle, has the stuff that makes him both an eminent physician and friend to his patients. His book will offer insight, hope, and understanding to its readers.

Michael Reese
Executive Director
King County Medical Society

Compassion, candor, and clarity characterize the writing of this book. I can identify with Dr. Johnson as a Christian, fellow physician, and former cancer patient.

Charles Setterstrom, M.D.
Grand Rapids, Michigan

This book will compel the patient with cancer to turn his heart toward God, who shows forth his lovingkindness in the morning and his faithfulness every night. Dr. Johnson encourages despairing cancer patients by reminding them that they have faith, hope, and love, which overcome sin, sorrow, and death.

Yu-Ming Chang, M.D.
Professor of Internal Medicine
Henan Medical University, China
Cancer Research Scientist
Memorial Sloan-Kettering Cancer Center

Dr. Johnson inspires cancer patients and provides us all with a healthy perspective. Most importantly, he reminds us that—with personal fortitude, faith, and modern medical technology—miracles happen!

Rudolf L. Brutoco, M.D., M.P.H.
President, LIFE-SAVERS FOUNDATION OF AMERICA

D0067656

To combat the fear experienced by cancer patients, Dr. Johnson has provided a complete crash course in cancer medicine. He also notes that "hope is a friend," and we share the understanding that all of our hope rests in the Lord.

> Mark G. Campbell, M.D.
> Cancer and Hematology Center
> Grand Rapids, Michigan

Dr. Johnson has given us tremendous insight into the often misunderstood world of cancer. His own personal experience will help every oncology patient on the journey toward "conquering cancer." This book is must reading for cancer patients, patients' families, and health care teams.

> Mark H. Kozakowski, D.O.
> Medical Missionary

As a practicing medical oncologist, I have seen the need for a book like *Conquering Cancer*. I think it should be required reading for people with cancer, people who have acquaintances with cancer, and people who treat cancer. There is something in this book for everyone.

> Ronald H. Lands, M.D.
> Medical Oncologist
> Oak Ridge, Tennessee

Conquering Cancer is an incisive, ambitious book on a complex subject. Dr. Paul Johnson succeeds in presenting this information in clearly understood terms. The chapter "You and Your Doctor" is superb and should be required reading for all patients—and my medical colleagues as well. It is easily worth the price of the book.

> Claude P. Ledes, M.D.
> Medical Oncologist
> Memphis, Tennessee

A compassionate physician tells how cancer can be challenged by a thorough understanding of the disease, a positive intellectual and spiritual approach, and the utilization of modern medicine. Not just for those with cancer, a wealth of information is presented in this book; this is a manual about hope.

John W. Riley III, M.D.
Associate Clinical Professor
University of Washington School of Medicine

This book is informative and helpful and offers realistic hope and personal encouragement to all cancer patients.

Aileen E. Denny, M.D.
Medical Oncologist
Brookfield, Wisconsin

Dr. Johnson's book is a helpful overview for those who wish to learn more about one of the most common—and dreaded—diseases of our time. Dr. Johnson approaches this disease as one who has fought cancer as a doctor, a patient, and a man of faith.

Fred Hardwicke, M.D.
Medical Oncologist
Arlington, Texas

Dr. Johnson adeptly approaches cancer from the clinical, scientific, and spiritual viewpoints, providing relevant information from each of these realms on the nature and process of cancer and its treatment.

Kenneth A. Feucht, M.D., Ph.D.
Chief Surgical Oncology
Keesler AFB Medical Center

Dr. Johnson has compiled a sensitive, personal, informative, and accurate resource that could be entitled, "Beating the Average." Only when we utilize our resources as a physician and patient team can this opponent, cancer, be beat. And win we will!

J. David Pitcher, Jr., M.D.
Orthopaedic Oncologic Surgery
Madigan Army Medical Center

Dr. Paul Johnson summarizes, in understandable terms, the array of conventional anticancer therapy and then treats us to his own experience of surviving cancer himself. The book is enlightening and well-balanced. It serves as a valuable companion to anyone dealing with cancer.

David E. Young, M.D.
Hematologist/Oncologist
Los Angeles, California

This is an excellent book for explaining to the cancer patient the process by which the cancer-treating team of physicians works together to provide curative treatment. It emphasizes a critical factor, which is an attitude of hopeful optimism based on the promises of Jesus Christ.

Calvin J. Dykstra, M.D.
Medical Oncologist
Grand Rapids, Michigan

Any cancer patient who reads this book will be struck by the author's obvious Christian perspective. The patient's diary section is the strongest part of the work—well-written, insightful, and extremely practical in terms of spiritual growth.

Charles Deur, M.D.
Arlington, Texas

CONQUERING CANCER

CONQUERING CANCER

An Invitation to Hope

Paul Johnson, M.D.

ZondervanPublishingHouse
Grand Rapids, Michigan

A Division of HarperCollinsPublishers

Conquering Cancer
Copyright © 1991 by Paul Johnson

Requests for information should be addressed to:
Zondervan Publishing House
1415 Lake Drive S.E.
Grand Rapids, Michigan 49506

Library of Congress Cataloging-in-Publication Data

Johnson, Paul, 1915–
    Conquering cancer : an invitation to hope / Paul A. Johnson.
        p. cm.
    Includes bibliographical references and index.
    ISBN 0-310-53781-9 (pbk.)
        1. Cancer—popular works. I. Title.
    RC263.J633 1991
    616.99′4–dc20   91–19799
                                                                                CIP

All Scripture quotations, unless otherwise noted, are taken from the HOLY BIBLE: NEW INTERNATIONAL VERSION (North American Edition). Copyright © 1973, 1978, 1984, by the International Bible Society. Used by permission of Zondervan Bible Publishers.

"The Road Not Taken" and "Acquainted with the Night" are from *The Poetry of Robert Frost*, edited by Edward Connery Lathem. Copyright 1928, © 1969 by Holt, Rinehart and Winston. Copyright © 1956 by Robert Frost. Reprinted by permission of Henry Holt and Company, Inc.

Permission has been granted to reprint a poem from *Caring Enough to Confront* by David Augsburger, © 1981, Regal Books, Ventura, CA 93003.

"Thank You for Waiting," by Ruth Harms Calkins is taken from *Tell Me Again, Lord, I Forget* (Elgin, Ill.: David C. Cook Publishing Co., 1974), p. 61. Used by permission.

Edited by Linda Vanderzalm
Cover design and illustration by Steve Allen

Printed in the United States of America

91 92 93 94 95 96 / AM / 10 9 8 7 6 5 4 3 2 1

CONTENTS

PART III
A Cancer Diary

A WORD FROM A CANCER SUFFERER

Dealing with the trauma of finding that you or a loved one must face a fight with cancer can be extremely difficult for any of us. In such circumstances, the peace a personal relationship with Jesus Christ provides cannot be exaggerated. However, we must individually accept certain responsibilities as we respond to hearing the words *tumor* or *cancer*. As a patient, or as a friend or loved one of a patient, the more we know about cancer the better we can assume our responsibilities in the fight against it.

In this excellent work, Dr. Paul Johnson provides a wonderful tool to help every victim of cancer more effectively battle that dreaded disease. The "victims" of cancer are not only those who discover that they have cancer, but also all of those close to them. The more all of us know about cancer and its treatment, the more we all can help and find hope.

Here you can find the help you need to understand that there is hope in the fight against cancer: hope that comes from wonderful technological advances and hope that comes from our Creator and our Savior, Jesus Christ.

> Dave Dravecky
> Former San Francisco Giants pitcher
> Author of *Comeback*

FOREWORD

The day I visited Dr. Paul in the hospital was also the first postsurgical day on which I received the shocking news that Paul was afflicted with a widespread malignancy, unrelieved by the surgical procedure. That day I thought that the solid foundation of my professional life and my very existence had been destroyed forever.

For over twenty years Paul's precious friendship and his ready professional support had been the sustenance and joy of my life as a physician. Just as Moses' tiring arm was held up by Aaron, so I always could obtain solace from Paul, who helped me make critical medical decisions. How could I face the future without Paul's ready succor?

Fortunately, with Paul's faith in God and the wise use of the available miracles of modern medicine, Paul made a spectacular and then almost unheard of recovery from a malignant disease, so that today he can share his past anxieties, his hopes, and his steadfast religious faith with thousands of troubled and suffering fellow members of humanity.

The many years of mutual trust and steady support have been inspirational to both of us.

Readers of these pages will be rewarded by the wisdom and comfort of Dr. Paul's message of hope.

> J. H. Lehmann, M.D.
> Past Chairman of the Board of Regents
> University of Washington

INTRODUCTION

Karl was a young family doctor who practiced in Bakersfield, California. He had worked hard and had established a growing practice because of his dedication and skill. People liked Karl, and he liked them.

Then in 1951, Karl noticed a tenderness in his right testicle. It quickly became more painful, inflamed, and swollen. He then developed a cough and low-grade fever. A chest X ray revealed shadows, and all too soon the diagnosis was confirmed. Karl had cancer of the testicle, and the cancer had metastasized, had spread to his lungs.*

The next two years were a nightmare for Karl, his wife (a pediatrician), and his two children. Karl had surgery. He took a series of radiation treatments which in reality destroyed everything in sight, including his bone marrow. He suffered anemia, weakness, periods of bleeding, loss of appetite, loss of weight, and all the other symptoms of radiation sickness.

One day Karl took his ten-year-old son to the local playing field to hit some baseballs for him to catch. On one weak swing, Karl fell to the ground. Two weeks later he began to bleed seriously and was taken to the hospital. His family was by his side as he slipped into a coma and died.

---

*I will explain most medical terms (like *metastasize*) the first time I use them in the book. If you happen to forget what a word means, check the index or the glossary of medical terms at the back of the book.

Karl was my brother. And that was in 1953. I share this story with you because if Karl had that same disease today, he would not have to die.

When I began practicing forty years ago, doctors knew almost nothing about cancer—except that people almost always died from it. Today that is simply not true. Today more people *survive* bouts with cancer than die from it.

That's why I have waited so long to write this book. I wanted to wait until I could be sure—medically sure—that when I offer you hope, it's not a false hope. And I wanted to be sure that you could understand just why you have hope.

Sometimes doctors are criticized for not explaining things to their patients. Too often the criticism is justified. We don't explain what a diagnosis means. We don't explain medical terms. We don't explain what is happening during treatment or why we prescribe a particular treatment. Personally I'm convinced that doctors *must* explain. A person who doesn't understand what is happening is going to be fearful and uncertain. And fear is one of recovery's greatest enemies. Our immune system, that complex, God-given system that enables our bodies to fight disease, can be crippled by fear and anxiety.

On the other hand, our immune system works best when we approach the future with confidence and hope. While fear is an enemy, hope is a friend. *Today you can have hope for a complete recovery from many cancers.*

I know how important hope is. In 1977, while I joked with a friend and his nurses who were doing a routine examination on me, I suddenly felt their silence. I watched as an orange-sized tumor took shape on the X-ray monitor. The form was unmistakable. I had a malignant lymphoma of the colon (a tumor of the lymph nodes).

I called my office and canceled the day's appointments.

Then I drove home to tell Genevieve, my wife. As I drove, I realized that everything had changed. I felt the fear you've known too if you've heard the words, "You have cancer." I felt the emptiness and the uncertainty. So I do understand.

I've also recovered, completely, from my cancer. I know how fresh and new life becomes when we realize we've been given another chance. And I want you to know that delight.

My desire in this book is to help you feel that someone is walking beside you as you fight against cancer. Although I address my thoughts especially to people who have cancer, I also think that people in close relationship to a cancer patient will find this book most helpful. In order to allay some of your fears, I've tried to provide as much information as possible to help you understand the process of diagnosing and treating cancer. For instance, Part I of this book describes in great detail what will happen to you at various stages of the discovery and treatment of your cancer. It includes hints for selecting a doctor. It includes a walk through a cancer surgery, a walk through radiation therapy, and a walk through chemotherapy treatments. It includes many helpful suggestions for maintaining physical, mental, and spiritual health during the treatment and recovery process.

Part II builds even more hope by helping you understand what makes normal cells turn into cancer cells, by describing how your body's immune system works toward your recovery, and how exciting medical advances lead to new and more effective forms of cancer treatment. Even though some of this section may seem a bit technical, I've tried to explain as clearly as possible the basic terminology and concepts that you will be encountering as you read the many articles about breakthroughs in cancer research and treatment. By understanding what these breakthroughs mean for you and your future, you can gain hope and confidence in conquering your cancer.

Part III is a cancer diary that I kept while I went through treatment for my colon cancer. The diary offers ninety "confidence builders"—including medical facts, real-life stories, thoughts from Scripture, a personal word or two—that can be used as daily readings to feed your mind and spirit with confidence and hope. I share it with you not so much as a definitive expression of what a person experiences while battling cancer but as an encouragement—an encouragement as you face feelings of disbelief, isolation, and uncertainty, and an encouragement for you to keep your own cancer diary.

This book is the best way I know how to do today what I've tried to do with such joy all my life: To help people conquer cancer.

To help you hope.

To help you recover.

To help you be well.

Paul A. Johnson
Seattle, Washington

PART I

You and Your Cancer

1

MODERN MIRACLES

Every so often I read a news item about a researcher's promise of some new miracle cure for cancer. I have to smile. What most people don't realize is that we already have a whole arsenal of "miracle cures" in today's fight against cancer.

When I started practicing medicine in the late 1940s, cancer was a complete mystery. A diagnosis of cancer meant almost certain death. We had no standard treatments, and many doctors relied on potions no better than the patent medicines of the 1800s. I remember how shocked I was when I took over the suburban Seattle practice of a very old doctor. People began coming in and asking for a refill of a mysterious syrup whose ingredients were known only to the old doctor and the pharmacist whose store was below my office. To order a refill, I had to know what was in the prescription, so I went down to see the pharmacist. He looked at me as if I were trying to steal the remedy!

What really amazed me, though, was the number of people who believed in the secret remedy and bristled if I questioned the merits of that magic potion. Yet I've seen this phenomenon happen often over the years. Where there's ignorance, there's room for soothsayers and quacks—even in the medical field, and especially with cancer. Countless people have promised magical "cures" that have no value whatsoever. In the 1950s, it was krebiozen, a chemical made in Illinois and endorsed by the noted physiologist Andrew Ivy. Later it was laetrile, a drug derived from apricot pits. You may be surprised to learn that the active ingredient in laetrile is the poison cyanide. The drug is now outlawed in the United States, but many people still go to Mexico to get it.

What hurts me is that today we have powerful medical weapons that really can help people conquer their cancer. While people chase after laetrile or some other magic cure, they waste vital time that could save their lives!

That really bothers me, particularly with cancer. My mother died of cancer. My older brother, who was my dearest friend, died of cancer. I fought my own battle with a deadly colon cancer thirteen years ago. Throughout my career as a physician and surgeon, combating cancer has been a deep, personal commitment. The last thing I want to see is anyone turn away from medicine's true modern miracles, to throw away his or her life by clutching desperately at some unproven miracle cure.

WHAT IS CANCER?

Cancer is the name given to a complex group of diseases that have certain things in common, the most important of which is the loss of control of cell division. Left to themselves, cancer cells will keep on replacing normal cells or multiplying and crowding out normal cells. Perhaps we can compare cancer to a weed that invades a flower garden. If the weed isn't removed, it will grow and multiply. Eventually the flowers will be choked out, and the weed will take over the garden.

In every healthy person, cells wear out and are replaced by other cells of the same kind. Liver cells die and are replaced by new liver cells that continue the function of the liver. Blood cells die and are replaced by new blood cells that take up their task in the body. But cancer cells are abnormal. They grow in an uncontrolled way. Though cancer cells replace and even kill normal cells in the liver or blood or in other organs, cancer cells do not function like liver cells or blood cells. When too many liver cells have been replaced, the liver fails—and the person dies. When too many cancer cells crowd into the intestines or into the lungs, these organs no longer function—and the person dies.

Some cancers are more aggressive than others, dividing and multiplying rapidly. They not only replace the organ where they originated, but they also invade nearby tissues, distorting and destroying wherever they go. Cancer cells also may travel through the blood or lymph systems and form colonies in distant sites. This spread of cancer beyond its original location is called *metastasis*.

Cancers are generally classified by the kind of tissues in which the uncontrolled cell growth originates. *Carcinomas* originate in tissues that cover a surface or line a body cavity; carcinomas are the most common type of cancer. *Sarcomas* originate in tissues that connect, support, or surround other tissues or organs. *Myelomas* are tumors made up of cells of the type normally found in the bone marrow. *Lymphomas* originate in the principle cells of the immune system called lymphocytes. They are distributed throughout the lymphatic network in the spleen, liver, thymus, bone marrow, and clusters called lymph nodes. *Leukemia* is a cancer of blood cells and blood-producing tissues.*

Unless the uncontrolled growth of cancer cells is checked, the person with cancer will die. Most doctors have seen cases in which the body's own defenses have overcome cancer, and the disease has simply gone away. These incidents of spontaneous remission do not happen often, however. To conquer cancer, you need to attack the cancer cells and purge them from the body. As you'll see later, we have three major weapons against cancer: surgery, which removes the cancer cells from the body; and radiation and chemotherapy, which attack the cancer cells while they are still in the body.

But the first and most vital thing to realize when you (or a loved one) have cancer is that *if you get to your doctor quickly and follow the therapy he or she prescribes,* you have a good chance to recover from most cancers. Many medical miracles are now available for your treatment.

DIAGNOSIS, THEN AND NOW

Before doctors can treat any disease appropriately, they must know what they're treating. Before doctors could talk intelligently about cancer or develop successful cancer treat-

---

*See the "Types of Cancer" chart in chapter 7, "On the Road to Recovery." This chart describes most cancers and gives basic information about their symptoms, growth patterns, seriousness, and other issues. If you have been diagnosed with a particular kind of cancer, you may want to check that chart now. Familiarizing yourself with the basic information about your cancer will help you sense which parts of the following chapters are particularly relevant to you.

ments, they had to describe and medically define each kind of cancer. When I began my medical career, the medical community had no commonly agreed on medical terminology to describe complex cancers. "Appendicitis" meant the same thing to doctors everywhere. But when it came to identifying and talking about cancers, different words might be used, not just in Boston and San Francisco, but within the same local community. Someone in Philadelphia might develop an effective treatment for one type of cancer and report it in a medical journal. But a doctor in Los Angeles might never realize the Philadelphia report related to cases he was treating.

In the mid-1970s, committees met to standardize descriptions of diseases to be used by all doctors everywhere and published a volume that indexed every type of disease and identified every complication. This book, known as *ICD-9-CM* (*International Classification of Disease-9th Edition-Clinical Modification*) is larger than the Bible and often much more difficult to understand. But today every disease has a code number, and in this day of the computer, it's all filed neatly on the office floppy disk. What's more, a frequently updated companion publication called *CPT* (*Current Procedural Terminology*) discusses the newest and most effective treatments for the diseases indexed in *ICD*.

What does this mean to the cancer patient? It means that today *every doctor* has access to the most up-to-date information about cancer types and treatments. You probably won't have to go to a hospital designated as a Cancer Center for diagnosis or treatment. Doctors who work with cancer patients in your area will be able to treat you effectively. What's more, if you have a complicated or unusual cancer, your doctors can phone the Cancer Information Service at the National Cancer Institute to receive a phoned-in computerized report that reviews state-of-the-art treatment for your specific type and stage of cancer. Or, even better, you can talk personally to one of the experts at a cancer center about your specific case.

The accurate, pinpoint definition of tumors is one of the most important modern cancer miracles. It has led to a literal explosion of accurate information about malignancies and their treatment. Today, with accurate diagnosis and a host of effective treatments, hundreds of thousands—no, millions—who suffer from cancer can expect to conquer it. The American Cancer Society's 1990 update estimates that 122 million Americans now living will have cancer sometime during their lifetimes. But because we now understand so much more about cancer, because we can diagnose tumors so much earlier and more accurately, and because we are rapidly developing more and more effective treatments, the great majority of those millions will survive their battle with cancer.

EARLY DIAGNOSIS

One of the most important weapons against cancer is early and accurate diagnosis. That's one reason why it's important to have regular medical checkups and to see a doctor immediately if you feel you have any of these familiar early warning signs:

- Unusual bleeding or discharge.
- A lump that doesn't go away.
- A sore that doesn't heal within two weeks.
- A change in bowel or bladder habits.
- Persistent hoarseness or cough.
- Indigestion or difficulty in swallowing.
- Change in a wart or mole.

Of course, none of these mean that a person *does* have

cancer. In most cases he or she won't. But the symptoms need to be checked by a doctor, who can make an accurate diagnosis.

Today it's rare to see a patient with a terminally advanced tumor. Take a person who notices some unusual rectal bleeding and follows the Cancer Society's advice to see a doctor. That bleeding may come from a small, less than one-centimeter polyp (a tiny growth). A doctor can remove that right in the office, under local anesthesia. The polyp is sent to the lab and examined by the pathologist. Most are noncancerous, and the treatment is over. But in a year or so that polyp might have become cancerous, and then treatment becomes complicated. If two or three years had passed, it would probably have been necessary to remove part of the bowel. Something as simple as today's early and proper treatment of a polyp is, to me, a giant step forward in our fight against cancer.

Or take another diagnostic tool, the Pap smear, which detects onset of cervical cancer. The test is a simple procedure: At a woman's regular gynecological checkup, the doctor simply scrapes the cervix, especially the opening (*os*) and gets enough cells to spread on a glass slide. These are sent to the laboratory, where a pathologist searches for abnormal cells. Since the Pap smear has been used regularly, the mortality rate from cervical cancer has nearly vanished! And all because the disease is treated in the early stage, before it has had a chance to get started.

In both of these illustrations diagnosis involved getting cells from a potentially cancerous area. The pathologist, who examines cells under a microscope to see if they are cancerous, must have tissues to work with. It's easy to get tissue from a rectal polyp or the cervix. But often the site of a possible cancer is hidden deep within the body. However, the use of the bronchoscope and laryngoscope—hollow, flexible tubes—allow doctors to see deep within the throat and lungs to retrieve pieces of tissue. Even more amazing is the laparoscope, a tube inserted through a very small incision at the navel. Using the laparoscope, doctors not only can see the tumors on ovaries, the uterus, and other areas, but they also can remove tissue from the tumor for further examination and diagnosis. Another amazing procedure enables doctors to insert an eight-inch needle into a tumor in the lung, liver, kidney, or other organ to obtain cells for examination. With the advent and regular use of these diagnostic tools, we can quickly and effectively, without the trauma of surgery, diagnose and define cancers—a vital step in their successful treatment.

But how do we locate tumors in order to know where to get tissue for examination? Modern medicine has an array of *imaging* tools that make it possible to see suspicious areas of cancerous growth deep within the body. Through the use of tools like the CT scan (computerized tomography, also known as a CAT scan [computerized axial tomography]), MRI (magnetic resonance imaging), and ultrasound, the medical community has been able to see strikingly clear, three-dimensional images of body organs, tissue, and tumors, allowing medical people to confirm the presence and extent of a cancer.

The use of a variety of dyes allow X rays to show features that would otherwise remain hidden. Barium studies (X rays taken of the upper or lower gastrointestinal tract as it is filled with a barium solution, which reveals on the X ray whether or not there are abnormalities) give us a window into the entire gastrointestinal tract. Through the use of intravenous pyelography (a process that allows doctors to view the kidneys and ureters), iodides are injected in the veins, making it possible to monitor the kidneys and ureters by X ray. If an area is suspicious, catheters (small tubes to allow fluids to be injected into or withdrawn from vessels or organs) are placed in from below and dye is injected for a more detailed study of the problem site. A cystoscope can be inserted the same way, for a visual inspection *inside* the bladder. Also the entire bilary system (the gall bladder, bile ducts, etc.) can be examined through the use of a contrast dye.

You don't need to try miracle diets or rely on alternative treatments to win your battle with cancer. What you do need to do is to rely on the real modern miracle: the medical treatment that is available everywhere in this country. With the help of skilled, caring doctors and nurses, you have the best chance in the world to conquer your cancer.

TREATMENT, THEN AND NOW

I mentioned that we have three basic weapons in today's fight against cancer: surgery, radiation treatments, and chemotherapy. The advances that have taken place in each area during my career are almost unbelievable.

Surgery

Surgery includes not only what goes on in the operating room, but in all the para-surgical areas, such as the recovery room, intensive care, and the surgical floor. Today's controlled atmosphere, with its specially trained nurses, is a far cry from what surgery was years ago, when the infection rate was high because of crude technique. The only antibiotics we had were sulfanilamide, sulfapyradine, and sulfathiozole—all had a very limited effect. Then came penicillin and the host of antibiotics that have followed.

The techniques of surgery itself have improved so that the

amount of trauma has consistently decreased. Operating time is shortened, and surgical judgment has improved. With controlled anesthesia, much more surgery can be safely performed. In the field of cancer we can do things now we would never have considered just ten years ago. Portions of livers can be removed, and large ovarian tumors can be excised, even though the cancer has spread. In certain cases, surgeons remove only the bulk of the tumor, trusting that chemotherapy can clean up the cancer that remains. What was thought terminal just ten years ago is no longer considered untreatable. Learn more about cancer surgery in chapter 3.

After a long and tedious cancer surgery, the patient goes to the recovery room. Under the skilled supervision of the anesthesiologist and specially trained nurses, the patient is carefully monitored for falling blood pressure, excess bleeding, blood gases, fluid and electrolyte balances, and the many things that are so vital to a good recovery. The nurses gathered around often remind me of mother hens guarding a little chick. The recovery-room staff keeps close watch until the patient is stable enough to take the next step, the intensive care unit. There a new group of nurses takes over, and the patient is hooked up to a whole battery of monitors. Vital signs are shown on a screen seen both at the bedside and at the nurses' station. Nurses also relieve much of the anxiety caused by fear of pain, offering the patient many options for pain relief.

Radiation

Radiation therapy is a second weapon against cancer. Fifty years ago, X-ray treatment was so crude and uncontrolled that far too many people died of radiation sickness. However, not only has the radiation equipment improved, but the manner in which the radiation is delivered has also improved—no guesswork, no random spraying of the body with harmful rays. The target and amount of radiation is fed into a computer and so directed that nearly all radiation is focused on the tumor itself. The maximum dose is delivered to the exact spot, sparing the normal tissue! Learn more about radiation therapy in chapter 4.

Not very long ago anyone getting radiation would end up with a severe skin burn, and often the treatment had to be interrupted because of the burn. Now, there is absolutely no evidence of skin change from radiation.

Perhaps the most amazing advance is a new source of radiation called a proton accelerator, which will provide much more power and accuracy in directing the radiation on the cancer without damaging healthy tissue. Each of these new machines costs at least $50 million. At present, the only facility using the proton accelerator available for patient care is in Loma Linda, California. While present radiation energy sources are adequate for the great majority of cancers, this new tool, to be in operation in 1991, provides stunning new capabilities.

A whole book could be written about such new technology alone. In fact, advances in technology are often featured in the media, because that's news, and good news at that. But we must be aware of one problem: Most advances—such as gene splicing, immunotechnology, and the proton accelerator—are reported as fact, even when in most cases they're theoretical or experimental (Part II will discuss some of these advances in greater detail). I do believe that total victory over cancer eventually will come through advances in molecular biology's growing understanding of the DNA, genes, and chromosomes (again, chapter 8 will define and explain DNA, genes, and chromosomes in more detail). One day we'll be able to prevent the whole complex of diseases known as cancer.

Chemotherapy

The third treatment for cancer is chemotherapy, which uses chemicals—drugs and hormones—to destroy cancer cells that can't be removed from the body.

Anyone who has been through chemotherapy knows it isn't easy. Some chemicals are worse than others, of course. But these are poisons—poisons to the cancer cells. Some people have serious side effects, while others have gone through long periods of treatment and had no side effects at all. But the bottom line is that today a wide range of chemicals that attack specific cancers are available. Learn more about chemotherapy in chapter 5.

But if you have cancer today, you want to hear about what will save your life now, not something that may work twenty years from now. The truly exciting news is that a whole host of medical and technological advances have led to a revolution in the war against cancer. We can treat cancer successfully right now. And the treatments are becoming more and more effective all the time. In fact, I'm alive only because of past technological breakthroughs that helped me conquer my own cancer! Because of these modern medical miracles already in place, I can honestly offer you hope.

THE MEDICAL TEAM

Today the medical community takes a team approach to treating cancer. The team is generally headed by a *primary-care physician,* who serves as a coordinator of the highly trained specialists who participate in your treatment. The primary-care physician will be your own doctor, the person who knows you and who has been your family's medical advisor. It's important for you to have a doctor whom you trust, who knows you as a person, and who will answer your questions and guide you through what may seem a maze of specialists and unfamiliar experiences.

The second important person on your team is a competent *oncologist,* a specialist trained in the causes, course, and treatment of cancer. This doctor is aware of the latest information about your specific type of cancer and the medical response to it. The oncologist will supervise your menu of chemotherapy, choose the chemical to be delivered, set frequency, and help you deal with any side effects. He or she will work closely with the primary-care physician in following your progress and will monitor you after recovery.

Next are the *radiologists,* both diagnostic and therapeutic. Diagnostic radiologists become more important all the time, because it is through their efforts that the progress of treatment is best monitored. Today, with ultrasound, MRI, and CT scans, along with other highly specialized scans, we can see in detail just what the tumor is doing and whether or not it has spread to other areas. Once the tumor has been assessed, the therapeutic radiologist uses X rays to kill the cancer cells.

The *surgeon* can also play an integral part of the team if surgical removal is an advised treatment. Here again your primary-care doctor will help you gain access to a qualified surgeon who can join the team and work with you.

The *pathologist* is another team member on whom the team leans for information about the cell structure of the tissue removed from your body. The pathologist not only determines whether the tissues are cancerous but also gives an informed opinion about the degree of malignancy and possible prognosis. After a surgical removal has been done, the pathologist is consulted to determine whether the entire tumor has been removed or whether some remains, needing follow-up chemotherapy, radiation, or both.

If I found anything unusual when I was doing surgery, I called the pathologist to the operating room. I wanted him or her to see the tumor in its viable form and anatomical relationships. The pathologist would point out exactly what tissue would be needed in the biopsy specimen. Many times I went with the pathologist to the lab to look at the "frozen section."

To prepare a frozen section, a pathologist freezes a piece of tissue with carbon dioxide until it is a cake of ice. He then shaves a very thin slice (about five microns thick) from the tissue, places it on a glass slide, stains it, and looks at it under the microscope. The pathologist can usually make a diagnosis on the frozen section.

The major advantages of the frozen section is that it takes only three minutes to prepare the slide for viewing, and if further surgery is indicated, it can be completed at that time with the same surgery team and anesthesia.

Because ice crystals damage the cell structure and the thickness of the slice of tissue distorts the details, a pathologist will always follow up with a "permanent section."

A permanent section takes eleven hours to prepare before it can be read under the microscope, and it is usually twenty-four hours before the doctor gets the pathologist's report. The permanent section is called "permanent" because the tissue is preserved in a paraffin block indefinitely without fear of deterioration.

The final people on the medical treatment team are the highly trained *nurses* and other hospital personnel who will care for the remaining treatment and recovery needs. When you view the entire team, you realize that they bring the knowledge and tools of many different medical disciplines to bear. And you realize they're there to help you conquer your cancer.

It's no wonder that the editor of *Prevention* magazine, Robert Rodale, wrote in the May 1989 issue of that magazine, "Start with quality medical care. Nothing—I repeat, *nothing*—matches the proven success rate of the medical treatments offered by the National Cancer Institute network. . . . Off-beat therapies often have little or no such evidence. So I would not forego a sure thing, whatever its drawbacks, to risk my life on a treatment with unknown effects."

WHEN REALITY STRIKES

I know from personal experience that cancer is the "dreaded disease." In my optimism in this chapter, I'm not trying to downplay the seriousness of anyone's diagnosis.

I remember the morning I went in for what I thought was a routine screening test. I was about sixty, so it was time to have an X ray of my gastrointestinal tract. No one expected to find anything. After all, I was going through this just because I had told my patients they should have screening tests, to let them know that what was good for them was good for me too. Much to the delight of the X-ray technicians, I went through all the tedious preparations of laxatives and cleansing enemas to prepare me for the barium enema examination. We joked and laughed together in an air of frivolity. The technicians had waited a long time to get me in this position!

Dr. Maxwell, the radiologist, proceeded with the exam, and everyone in the room could see the monitor, which is nothing but a television-like screen. As the barium made its way up my colon, at about eighteen inches, it clearly outlined a mass about the size of an orange. We all saw it at the same time.

Now, an orange-sized tumor of the colon is gigantic. It got oppressively quiet in the room, and Dr. Maxwell kept moving the equipment to scan other areas of my colon, only to sneak back from time to time to see if the tumor was still there. It was.

I can't explain just what my reaction was. I had had no symptoms and this came as a complete surprise to all of us. Any remnant of frivolity disappeared. It was crunch time.

The strange thing was, I felt like getting dressed, going to the office, and forgetting the whole thing. After all, I felt fine. If I became enmeshed in my routine for the day, maybe the whole thing would go away. As I was dressing, I tried to get my thoughts together. I knew the first order of business was to tell my wife, Genevieve. So I drove home, with my mind buzzing the whole time. When I got there, Genevieve knew that something was wrong. I never came home at that time of day. And I had to tell her.

I had gone through cancer with my mother and my brother. Now it was my turn.

It's different when it's your own body.

So please believe me. I'm not making light of cancer. Not at all. I understand your doubts and fears because I've felt them. But I also know that it's worth meeting cancer head on.

I've fought cancer and won.

I've seen the amazing advances medicine has made in the treatment of cancer in the past forty years.

I've seen hundreds of my own patients fight cancer and win.

Because of these things, I want you to face your own cancer with a sense of confidence and of hope. Go to your doctor. Get the truly outstanding medical treatment available today.

In the rest of this book I'll try to help you understand the three cancer treatments better. I'll try to help you make some of the critical decisions that will give you significant control in your battle with cancer. And I'll keep on giving you reasons to have *hope,* whatever kind of cancer you need to conquer.

QUESTIONS FOR THOUGHT
OR GROUP DISCUSSION

1. What were your feelings when you or your loved one was diagnosed with cancer?
2. What were some of the ideas you had about cancer and its treatment? Make a list and compare your list with the ideas others have or have had.
3. Which of your ideas about cancer are supported by this chapter? Which of your ideas may be wrong?
4. List at least three reasons why you can feel more hopeful about the possibility of recovering from cancer.
5. What questions do you have about your cancer? List them. As you read through this book, look for answers to those questions. If at the end of your reading, you still have questions, take them to your doctor.

2

YOU AND YOUR DOCTOR

Not too long ago, having cancer marked a person as "inferior." A cancer patient felt a sense of guilt and tried to conceal the disease. The disease was embarrassing and almost seemed to demand quarantine. The social stigma associated with cancer actually prevented many people from seeking early attention from their doctor.

Today, through education, this attitude has slowly changed. Cancer is no longer an indictment. While cancer is no longer a secretive disease, it still generates fear and many other painful emotions. I know some of the feelings I had when I was diagnosed with colon cancer, even though I was fully aware of the resources available for my treatment. I was startled because I had had no warning. I felt alone. I felt lost. I tried pretending nothing was wrong. I asked, "Why me, Lord?" That taste of self-pity was spoiled when I heard the answer echo in my mind. "Why *not* me?"

The fact is that anyone can have cancer. And anyone with cancer will experience a variety of nagging, uncomfortable feelings. Some of the most common emotional reactions have been collected in a thick paperback called *Choices,* written by Marion Morra and Eve Potts (Avon, 1987). The authors list the following reactions and suggest that cancer patients check off those they feel most intensely.

1. Terror. "I don't want to die." And, "I'm afraid."

2. Denial. "I can't believe this is happening to me." "Maybe it will all go away." And, "It couldn't be cancer because no one in my family ever had cancer."

3. Emptiness. "I feel as if I've been thrown off a cliff."

4. Isolation. "This is the loneliest experience of my life." And, "No one else can know how I feel."

5. Uncertainty. "If it really is cancer, what will it do to my life?" And, "What if the doctor says I have to go to the hospital right away?"

6. Indecision. "I don't know how to tell my family." And, "People will treat me differently if they find out I have cancer."

7. Dread. "I'm going to be in a lot of pain." And, "I don't want to lose my lung (or breast or leg)."

8. Self-pity. "Why me? Why couldn't it have been someone else?"

Interestingly enough, emotional reactions frequently don't match the seriousness of the diagnosis. I've seen patients with the most serious tumors battle their cancer with unfailing good humor and optimism, while others diagnosed with a truly minor cancer simply fall apart.

During my years of practicing medicine, I've had a firsthand opportunity to observe many people at close range. I soon realized that a primary-care doctor must assume many roles. What cancer patients need is a skilled physician who is also a friend, counselor, confessor, and advisor. In other words, cancer patients need a therapeutic relationship with their doctor. Treating the body just isn't enough. In fact, it's difficult to treat the body if patients continue to be anxious, fearful, and insecure. Practicing medicine is an art that calls for personal involvement with patients in addition to a skilled application of medical technology. A caring, therapeutic relationship with a skilled physician will reduce a patient's fears and make a vital contribution to recovery.

WHAT EVER HAPPENED TO THE FAMILY DOCTOR?

Before World War II, every family had a doctor who took care of all their medical problems. That doctor was a trusted advisor, someone who was always available. A few specialists did practice medicine, but they were called in only unusual cases. The family doctor could take care of eighty to ninety percent of a family's medical problems. That system had its advantages as well as its disadvantages. Medical technology was in its infancy then, and diagnoses were made on signs and symptoms. The doctors of those days became astute at diagnosing and treating with very little help. The family doctor became an integral part of every family's experience and was almost revered. Patients had that sense of closeness so important in a therapeutic relationship.

After the war, as the doctors returned home, only a few went back to family practice. The day of specialization had dawned. Family practice was too demanding, and the hours were too long. Besides, specializing brought prestige and often paid more money. Medical technology advanced rapidly, and doctors needed more training to stay on the cutting edge. But the attraction of specialization drained the supply of doctors available for families and their common problems. That drain has never been stopped, and today the vacuum created is filled by others who list themselves as primary-care physicians: internists, obstetricians, gynecologists, even surgeons, as I was. But the "family doctor" of the past is gone.

If you have a suspicious problem that you think might be cancer, you need to turn to a doctor in whom you have confidence, someone who can take the role of friend as well as physician, someone who will be sensitive to your feelings as well as your physical symptoms, someone who will give comfort and support. You may be able to find a primary-care physician who practices family medicine. If not, choose an internist or other specialist who knows you and with whom you've had previous contact. This will be the doctor who makes the initial diagnosis and leads you into some very important decisions. It's imperative to develop this initial relationship with someone who helps you feel secure.

The key to the therapeutic relationship is good communication. Since retiring from practice, I do public relations work for the King County Medical Society. In fielding questions about health care and health problems, I frequently discover that a major problem is the lack of communication between doctor and patient. I have to admit that the doctor is usually the problem. For one reason or other the doctor doesn't adequately explain what is going on inside the patient's body. As a result patients are left with misconceptions, feelings of alienation, fear, and even suspicions. Believe me, you don't want this to happen in your fight against cancer. *You need a skilled doctor who cares—and who communicates.*

If you are diagnosed with cancer by a general practitioner whom you've just begun to see and whom you don't know well, he or she usually will refer you to a specialist: an oncologist, a surgeon, or a radiologist, depending on the kind of cancer you have. When this happens, the specialist will then become the coordinating physician, and he or she has to be your advocate. The specialist has to be the one who keeps in close touch with you, who keeps you informed, who guides you to make good decisions, who helps you feel comfortable—in short, the person who communicates constantly with you. *It is vitally important that you feel comfortable with the doctor who directs your cancer treatment.*

WHAT TO LOOK FOR IN YOUR DOCTOR

It's true that many doctors aren't good communicators. But you still can find a doctor with whom you can have a truly therapeutic relationship. Here are some of the traits I suggest you look for in the physician who is to direct your cancer treatment.

1. Choose a doctor who is well respected by colleagues. Competent doctors gain the respect of their colleagues. This is reflected in several things. They have staff privileges at the first-class hospitals of the city. They are active in the staff administration of at least one major institution.

This may sound strange, but a number of doctors don't have good judgment. In our hospital, I was in the operating rooms nearly every day and was able to see what was going on. It was easy to observe the work of the various surgeons. It became evident to both doctors and nurses which surgeons did the good surgery and which did the questionable. A surgeon could have good skills, but he or she may not have had the necessary good judgment about when to operate and how much surgery to do. The tendency was to operate too often and to do too much. To control the quality of medical care, the hospital established a committee that reviewed all of the cases done in surgery and discussed them with the surgeons who were responsible. As a result of the continual internal review, offending surgeons were under tight scrutiny and were controlled as to what they could or could not do.

The point I'm making is that staff or key review-committee membership is a sign that a doctor is well respected by his or her colleagues. And this is a real confidence builder for any patient.

2. Choose a doctor who communicates and explains things well. Nothing produces as much anxiety as a doctor who does not explain. Before long your imagination starts running in high gear, and you suspect the worst. Your doctor should take time to make clear just what your symptoms and the diagnosis mean. The doctor should explain what you're up against and what your options are. Step-by-step explanation of what is happening and why is vital. Make sure your doctor has good communication skills and is willing to take time to answer your questions.

3. Choose an experienced doctor who takes your symptoms seriously. I remember one middle-aged man who came in to see me because he was tired and had lost weight. His appetite was poor, but he blamed that on the fact that his business wasn't doing well and he had been under heavy stress. He had had a hard time sleeping for the past two weeks and had night sweats. Otherwise, he had no other symptoms. He just didn't feel well. And, oh yes, he was losing interest in his work and even in golf, his special outlet for stress.

When I saw him, he really didn't look very healthy. His color was sallow, and his face sagged. I thought for sure I would find something during the physical examination, but everything looked normal. The lab work showed a slight anemia and increased sedimentation rate of the red blood cells, both consistent with a smoldering disease. The chest X ray was normal.

It would have been easy to dismiss his symptoms as nothing serious, but I couldn't do that. He returned to the office a week later, no better. He continued to lose weight and feel weak, though he still felt no pain. I consulted with my partner, who examined him and found no abnormal test results.

Then we decided to consult with our radiologist and ask for any help he could give us with his high-tech imaging devices. This patient was a real challenge for us because we were concerned that he might have a malignant tumor that was very difficult to pinpoint. We couldn't let him go without going over him thoroughly. We had to find the cause of his symptoms.

This is the kind of case that drives doctors crazy and causes them to lie awake nights, going over all the findings and planning what to do the next morning to throw light on the diagnosis. We doctors discussed the case in the staff room while the radiologist planned tests to pinpoint the problem. He was convinced we were going to find a tumor in the abdomen and set out to locate it by means of a CT scan. He went over the abdomen, organ by organ, and finally found the tumor, in an almost impossible area to diagnose. There it was: a suspicious area in the tail of the pancreas. By the time that tumor would have been large enough to feel through the abdominal wall, it would have been too late to do anything. But now it was early. We discussed the whole thing with the patient and his wife. During surgery two days later, we found the malignant tumor, well contained and easy to remove. We found no evidence of spread. Cancer of the pancreas is notoriously bad, but with the aid of the radiologist and his equipment, we removed the cancer in time.

4. Choose a doctor who is available. The minute a doctor starts treating a patient, he or she accepts a great responsibility. Some shoulder it better than others. Your doctor needs to be available to care for you and answer your questions, whether or not it's an emergency. Even though your doctor may not be in his or her office when you need some advice or information, the doctor's staff will be able to make contact with him or her.

5. Choose a doctor who cares. I can honestly say that my partner and I never let commercialism influence the way we practiced. We loved people, and that was easy for our patients to see and feel. When you find a qualified doctor who cares, you can confidently commit yourself into his or her care.

6. Choose a doctor who respects your rights. During the course of cancer treatment many decisions will need to be made, and you must be included in every one. You have the right to accept or refuse any test or treatment that is suggested. And before any final decision is made, you have a right to ask the medical people involved to discuss and clarify with you all the available options. You may want to consult another expert before acting on a proposed test or treatment. You even should be included in the decisions that aren't that important. With that in mind, choose a doctor who shows a willingness to have you participate in every decision and who will carefully discuss each choice with you.

7. Choose a doctor whose office staff is friendly and professional. An office staff typically reflects the doctor who employs it. If the staff seems harried and disorganized or is short and uncommunicative with you, the doctor will usually have these same traits. On the other hand, if the staff seems well organized, relaxed, and willing to take time to answer your questions, the doctor probably will be like this too. Besides, you will usually have to go through the office staff to reach your doctor. So you definitely want to feel they're on your side and will do everything they can to help.

8. Choose a doctor who has a sense of humor. This qualification may at first seem trivial in the context of facing a life-threatening illness. But a person who can help you keep perspective and break the seriousness of your treatment will be an invaluable aid in your fight against cancer.

After spending a couple of weeks with the technicians who were giving me radiation treatment, I felt comfortable with them. At one point they had to mark the position of my kidneys and liver by painting diagrams of them, kidneys on my back and liver on my abdomen. My teasing of the technicians had caught up with me, and they had a field day body painting my liver and kidneys. We laughed through the whole treatment.

9. Choose a doctor who radiates optimism. One of your first reactions to the diagnosis of cancer probably will be, What are my chances of recovery? There may be a statistical answer—but it is probably wrong.

I remember the day the nation learned that President Reagan had colon cancer. When the medical spokesperson was asked about the prognosis, he stated that President Reagan had a fifty-percent chance of living for five years. I was on the air myself that day, doing my regular medical radio program in Seattle, and naturally the moderator wanted to talk about the president's condition. I pointed out the fallacy of putting all our confidence in a set of statistics. That fifty-percent figure was a group prediction and included all kinds of people: those who smoked and drank heavily, those who had bad eating habits, and those with all sorts of unhealthy lifestyles. Here was the president, who radiated exceptionally good health, had excellent health habits, who exercised daily, and had a great attitude. That "average" just didn't apply to him. He had every expectation of beating the average—and he did! The only thing statistics do is suggest how serious a cancer may be. They do not predict whether or not *you* will recover. Your doctor should point that out and help you work optimistically toward becoming one of those who do get well.

10. Choose a doctor with a pleasant personality. You need to feel at ease when talking to your doctor. You'll quickly sense whether your personalities mesh and whether he or she is concerned about making you comfortable and relaxed. During any long-term cancer treatment, a person experiences many ups and downs. It's a great encouragement to know your doctor cares about you personally and has time to talk with you about your treatment. Perhaps the best way to say this is, choose a doctor whom you would like as a friend.

Many cancers take a combination of treatments, such as surgery followed by chemotherapy, followed by radiation. All that takes time and can extend well over a year. During that year you'll experience ups and downs and probably want to quit treatment in the middle if you experience side effects. During this time you'll need to feel close to the doctor in whom you have the greatest confidence. He or she will have a vital role in keeping your spirits up and in helping you maintain hope. You really will need to choose a doctor with whom you can have a healing, positive, therapeutic relationship.

Having considered all these qualities, what if you don't feel comfortable with the doctor directing your treatment or one of the specialists working with you? If you become so uneasy that the relationship is seriously bothering you, you need to change doctors. If you are having trouble with a specialist, go back to your primary-care doctor and ask him or her to recommend a replacement. That happened to me when I was treated for my cancer. My oncologist was competent, but he was cold. It depressed me just to see him. And I sure didn't need anything more to depress me just then! So I did just what I advise you to do. I changed doctors.

If you decide you must change doctors, don't feel as if you have to explain why you've chosen to leave a doctor's care. You don't need the stress of a face-to-face meeting. If you feel you need to explain, send the doctor a brief explanatory note.

WHAT WILL YOUR DOCTOR
WANT FROM YOU?

Let me answer this question by describing how I would deal with you if you were my patient. Once I had the pathology report with a firm diagnosis proven by biopsy, I would call you in for a consultation, asking you to bring along a person close to you—your spouse, a parent, a close friend—a person who will see you through the process of treatment.

When you arrive, the three of us go into my inner office to discuss the entire situation. We look at all the facts and feelings, questions and answers. The third person is there to hear what is said and to help you digest the entire encounter.

I say encounter, for that's what it is. We must try to form a partnership so that we can work effectively together to proceed with the treatment. This sense of partnership in the battle is one of the most important elements of the doctor-patient relationship.

I believe in telling you everything I know about your particular case and about the kind of cancer you're up against. The more we can identify with each other, the more comfortable we both are during the course of treatment. I then proceed to explain the cancer, how extensive it is, the positive and negative qualities of this particular kind of cancer, and how these qualities affect you. I explain the available treatments and how we can approach the treatment process.

Together we set some goals. If surgery is involved, we plan the time for the surgery, how long you will be in the hospital, what will be done with alternatives if necessary. I try to cover all the things that might happen and then answer your questions. If no surgery is involved, I introduce you to the oncologist who will be directing your chemotherapy or the radiologist who will be directing your radiation therapy. Before the end of the consultation, I try to develop a trust relationship. I offer my time and advice any time, at your request. I spend a lot of time building a comfort zone for both of us.

Our time together is completely uninterrupted. Before the

consultation began, I asked my staff to make sure no phone calls or staff reports would disturb us. I want you to feel that during our time together, you are the most important person in my life. I will probably tell you a bit of my own story of conquering cancer, helping you know that I understand, that your concerns are my concerns. I want to convince you that I care and that this isn't just another routine case for me.

What do I as a doctor want from you in this relationship? I want your trust. I want you to ask all your questions and share your fears. Treating cancer can be a long-term commitment, and I want you to feel you can trust me. I want you to know that you can ask any questions and expect an honest answer.

A healthy doctor-patient relationship is more important in cancer treatment than in the treatment of most other diseases. I can look back at my cases and see many cancer patients who have become lifelong friends. Most of them are people who were extremely sick and had to trust me with tough decisions.

What I want as a doctor, then, is really just what you want. A close relationship. A partnership. A willingness to share with me what you are feeling, what you are experiencing, what you are going through. I want that because I'm a healer, not just a technician. I want it because I know that building and maintaining that kind of relationship will provide the best context in which you can conquer your cancer.

One patient I remember well is Henry. Henry was a doctor shopper, and he had seen a lot of them. His problem was abdominal pain. Like several other patients of mine, his eating habits were poor. He drank too much alcohol, especially while he traveled. And he became fatigued easily and didn't feel rested after a night's sleep. Henry had climbed the success ladder with the railroad and was in a responsible position.

YOU AND YOUR DOCTOR

When Henry came into the office, he carried on a loud, rapid-fire conversation with the receptionist. I learned from talking to this brusque man that he had received most of his medical care in railroad hospitals, for which he had no respect. But in the last ten years he had had six operations on his stomach, and his intestine was still not well. I could see that he entirely trusted technology. He had no doubt that modern medicine could cure him while he continued on his job. He thought of his body as he thought of one of his locomotives: If it's broken, fix it.

I tried to explain to him that the human body was different from a machine, but this didn't sink in. When I asked him why he thought the other surgeries didn't help him, he replied, "I just went to the wrong roundhouse!"

Henry's perspective was wrong. We're not just machines. The human body is far more than a mechanical contraption; it is a complex interaction of systems and cells that form part of a larger whole. When treating any serious disease—especially cancer—we have to deal with the whole person. Treating your whole person—your diseased body, your feelings, your fears, your spirit, your mental health—is one of your doctor's most important roles.

The good news is that you will find many doctors who will fill this role with competence and care. Oh, you won't hit it off with every doctor. And some people will be totally comfortable with a doctor that you just can't feel close to. But when you find a doctor with whom you feel secure and safe, you've definitely moved ahead in your fight to conquer your cancer.

QUESTIONS FOR THOUGHT
OR GROUP DISCUSSION

1. What positive impact of a good doctor-patient relationship have you experienced? What negative impact of a poor doctor-patient relationship have you felt? How has either affected you or your loved one during the course of treatment?

2. How do you feel about the doctor now guiding your own or your loved one's cancer treatment? Rank each item from "1" (lowest) to "5."

The doctor is competent	1	2	3	4	5
The doctor takes time to explain	1	2	3	4	5
The doctor answers my questions	1	2	3	4	5
The doctor explains options and helps me make informed choices	1	2	3	4	5
The doctor is someone I like and feel confidence in	1	2	3	4	5

What does the pattern of your evaluation (above) suggest about your relationship to your present doctor?

3. If you don't have confidence in your doctor, what do you plan to do about it? One cancer researcher with whom I consulted said that spontaneous remissions of cancer (recovery without treatment) take place in about 1 of 500 or 1 of 1000 cases. Pretty poor odds! If you don't feel confident in your doctor, *don't* stop treatment. Get another doctor. Which of the suggestions for choosing a doctor seem most important to you?

3

WHAT TO EXPECT FROM SURGERY

Right now I'm watching a good friend die.

He could have avoided his whole crisis.

He developed a basal-cell carcinoma (a skin cancer of the innermost cells of the deeper epidermis) on the top of his head. He is bald, and the lesion (the diseased area) was easy to see and follow. But my friend is the type who never quite gets around to taking care of something so trivial. He had no pain, and the sore was so small that he never found time to interrupt his routine to take care of himself. The days of neglect grew into weeks, the weeks into months. By the time he got around to making an appointment with his doctor, the lesion was an inch wide with raised, pearly borders. And it had an ulcer in the center. He also had some enlarged lymph nodes behind his ear on one side.

By not seeing a doctor and by allowing the prime time to pass, my friend had converted a simple problem to a very complex one, for the cancer had spread into the lymphatics, making it impossible to be removed entirely by surgery. He now could receive only other, less effective treatment.

Today my friend's tumor is beyond the boundaries of containment and has spread inward to who knows where. Radiation was recommended as his only chance of treatment, but his inaction had lowered his expectation of cure to less than twenty-five percent. During the course of radiation, he quit the treatments. His reason was that it "wasn't doing any good." Today there is virtually no hope he will be cured, and his tumor is growing merrily on its way.

I know that many people are frightened by the thought of even simple surgery. But the scalpel in the hand of a skilled surgeon isn't an enemy. It is often your very best friend, a life-saving friend. If your cancer is diagnosed early—if you don't dawdle and let precious time slip away before seeing the doctor—and if your cancer can be removed by surgery, you have a good chance of conquering the disease.

However, everyone has the choice. You can pretend the problem isn't there, as my friend did. You can even refuse a treatment that is known to be successful. A patient has the final say in his or her case. But my friend found out that there's a price to pay for the wrong choice. And, unfortunately, he is paying it.

The purpose of this chapter is to help you look ahead to the possibility of surgery. I want to help you understand what's involved in both simple and more complex surgeries. And I hope I can quiet any of your hidden fears, which keep some people from choosing surgery when their medical team recommends it.

WHAT TO EXPECT FROM SURGERY

WHY RECOMMEND SURGERY?

The goal of every responsible cancer treatment is *to get rid of cancer cells* that have been found in the body. As we have mentioned before, that can be done in two basic ways: cutting out the cancerous tissue (surgery) or killing the cancer cells while they are still in the body (radiation and/or chemotherapy). Frequently a combination of treatments works best.

For instance, a cancer may first be treated surgically, attempting to remove as much as is possible and safe. What remains of the cancer is then treated with radiation, chemotherapy, or a combination of the two. Sometimes all of a tumor can't be removed by surgery because the cancer cells are so close to nerves or a critical organ that surgery would not be safe. In general, a surgery that can remove all the cancer in the body is preferred over other treatments. Remember, early diagnosis is important here. If a cancer can be caught while it's still localized, before it has spread to other parts of the body, complete surgical removal is often possible.

Before any doctor recommends surgery, he or she will carefully *grade* and *stage* your tumor, using a standard classification system that has been developed in the past twenty-five years. This classification involves defining both the type of cancer cells involved (grade) and the extent or spread (stage) of your cancer.

Grades of Cancer

Cancers are classified into four grades of cells. A grade-1 tumor contains cells that are highly differentiated. This means that the cell structure resembles the cells from the site of your tumor (stomach, muscle, liver, skin, etc.). In general, the more differentiated a tumor is, the less malignant it is, but it is also less likely to respond to treatment. However, if the surgeon is able to remove this cancer, he or she probably will be able to remove it all.

Grade 4, at the other end of the classification system, is highly undifferentiated. We call it *anaplastic*. A grade-4 tumor has few characteristics of the cells at the site where it developed. This cancer grows faster than a grade-1 tumor. It also has a tendency to spread more rapidly to other sites in the body. Because the cells are undifferentiated, it is also difficult to tell whether the place the cancer was found is the original site. But the good news is that while grade-4 cancer grows rapidly, it also responds well to treatment.

Stages of Cancer

Stages classify the extent or spread of a cancer. A stage-1 cancer is contained and hasn't left its original site; it hasn't spread at all. A stage-2 cancer has invaded surrounding structures, such as fat or muscle. A stage-3 cancer has reached lymph nodes in the immediate region. A stage-4 cancer has spread through the lymphatic system or blood system to distant organs. This is a general classification of stages and is not always applicable to all forms of cancer.

Before recommending surgery to treat your cancer, the medical team will review all of the information about your tumor and its characteristics as recorded in your chart. This information includes the history of the cancer, the physical findings, the biopsy report by the pathologist, the laboratory results, and the imaging reports, such as X rays, CT, MR, or ultrasound scans. Everything about you, the patient, is brought to the conference table. Sometimes a pre-operative biopsy is not possible, but if it is, the report will be very helpful. For example, the diagnosis of cancer of the breast is confirmed only by the pathologist who identifies cancer cells.

Surgery would not be considered unless the pathologist reported cancer cells in the specimen.

WHAT SHOULD I KNOW ABOUT THE RECOMMENDED SURGERY?

Surgery is scary, even when you trust the doctor who recommends it. While you don't want to dawdle, as my friend did, you don't need to jump into surgery like a youngster jumping off the diving board—with your eyes shut, desperately holding your nose.

I never felt threatened when my patients wanted a second opinion before going ahead with surgery. That's the advantage of modern medicine. If you want a second opinion, ask your doctor to provide the consultant with all of the information on the chart. Then the consultant's opinion will be based on the entire case study, and the independent confirmation will make you feel a lot better about your surgery. If questions are raised, talk them over with your original doctor and totally satisfy yourself that you are on the right course and are in competent hands. If you are not completely comfortable, you should make a change.

But before you decide on surgery, you will want to ask your doctor several questions. Asking questions doesn't mean that you're challenging your doctor's medical ability. Asking questions means that you want to know everything you can learn about your surgery so that you can make an informed decision and can feel as comfortable as possible with your operation. The more you understand about the reason for your surgery and about how the operation will affect you, the more confident you'll feel. That sense of calm assurance, that conviction that this is the right thing makes a big difference in how quickly you'll recover from your operation.

What, then, are some of the questions you may want to ask when your doctor proposes surgery? The following list suggests a number of reasonable questions that will help give you peace of mind.

QUESTIONS TO ASK YOUR SURGEON

What do you expect the surgery will achieve?

Exactly what will you do when you operate?

How many times have you performed this operation?

What will happen if I don't have the surgery?

What are the risks involved in the surgery?

How do the benefits outweigh the risks?

What tests will I have to take when I enter the hospital?

What else will happen before the surgery?

How long will I have to be in the hospital?

How will I feel after surgery?

How will you control any pain?

What symptoms should I report to you after the surgery?

Will the surgery have any negative long-term effects?

How long will it be before I can get back to my work/home?

How much will all this cost?

WHAT TO EXPECT FROM SURGERY
WALKING THROUGH A CANCER OPERATION

I've spent a lot of my professional life in operating rooms. I became very comfortable in that setting; it almost became my second home. Working closely with a skilled team that included my partner, operating-room nurses, an anesthesiologist, and a pathologist was a deeply rewarding experience.

Cancer surgery has become much more satisfying as well. It's so much safer than when I started. And we can do things today that we wouldn't have considered just twenty-five years ago: removing lungs, lobes of livers, and portions of pancreases, for example. Surgeries done in our country are done in high-tech medical environments. Even the simple things have become mechanized. A blood count, for example, is done automatically by computers and special instruments. Today monitors and printouts describe the state of the patient every moment. We know the different arterial and venous pressures, the blood gases, the electrical waves of the heart muscles, brain waves, pulmonary pressures. You name it, we can measure it. The net result is that a patient is much safer traveling through the critical hours during and after an operation.

I realize that the same operating room that feels so friendly and familiar to me is going to feel strange to you. The maze of tubes and machines is confusing and probably frightening as well. But perhaps I can help you feel more comfortable by describing a cancer operation.

Let's walk through a typical colon-cancer surgery recommended for Jim. As we follow Jim through the process, you'll better understand what happens in surgery and perhaps feel more comfortable about having an operation yourself.

The Decision

I meet with Jim and his wife and explain everything we've discovered about his cancer. I recommend surgery and explain my reasons, making it clear that Jim has rights. He has a choice. But I tell him plainly that in my opinion surgery is his best chance for a cure. I also outline a treatment schedule— the steps I think we need to take and the time frame we need to work in. After this consultation Jim and his wife go home and talk it over. The next day Jim calls back. He's decided to go ahead with surgery, and he wants to get it over as soon as possible.

Preparing for the Operation

I (or my office staff) call the hospital and arrange a time for the operation. I make arrangements to insure that Jim's colon will be completely cleansed for the surgery: I instruct Jim to have a clear, liquid diet for three days before hospitalization and instruct the hospital staff to order laxatives and enemas.

Jim is admitted to the hospital the day before the scheduled surgery. Shortly after Jim is admitted, the floor nurse carries out my order, "Enemas until crystal clear." The nurses kid me about those orders, calling me "the crystal kid." But it really helps the surgery and the post-operative process to have a spotlessly clean colon. It reduces the danger of infection, and it helps Jim recover his bowel function after surgery.

The night before surgery Jim takes a shower, and his abdomen is cleansed again with soap and water. His excess hair is removed, and he is seen by the doctor who will give the anesthesia. That doctor goes over Jim's medical history, examines his heart and lungs, reviews his lab tests, and then explains what will be done in the morning. He or she usually orders some medication that will help Jim sleep. I see Jim once more that night and check to see that everything is in order.

In the Operating Room

In the early morning, the nurse gives Jim his pre-op medicine. This consists of something to relieve his anxiety and something else to dry up the bronchial secretions caused by the anesthetic. An orderly transfers Jim to a gurney (a wheeled cart), covers him with a blanket, and takes him to the surgery suite and the operating room, where the anesthesiologist whom Jim met the previous night greets him.

A nurse inserts a catheter into Jim's bladder and runs its tube into a bottle on the floor. The catheter will keep Jim's bladder empty during the surgery, will let the surgeon have a better view of the pelvic portion of the abdomen during the operation, and will prevent injury to the bladder during the operation.

Another nurse carefully inserts into Jim's arm a needle linked by a long clear tube to a bottle of liquid. The anesthesiologist will inject medication into this IV (intravenous) tube, from which the medication will flow into Jim's vein. Soon Jim is asleep.

A number of precautions are taken to protect Jim from exposure to bacteria or other substances that could cause complicating infections. All the people in the room wear light-green shirts and pants, hats over their hair, sterile paper boots over their shoes, and masks on their faces.

The circulating nurse prepares Jim's abdomen, scrubbing it with soap and water and applying an antiseptic solution. The scrub nurse then drapes the abdomen and completes the work of arranging sterile instruments on a sterile table.

All instruments used in the surgery have been previously sterilized in the hospital's pressure-steam autoclaves, which kill not only bacteria but also spores, which are bacteria's defense against heat. In addition, an indicator is placed inside every pack of instruments when it's sterilized. On unwrapping the pack, the indicator must have changed color. If that doesn't happen, the contents of the pack are not sterile, and the surgeon will not use the instruments.

About this time my partner, Dr. Eddy, and I come into the operating room. The two of us have assisted each other in surgery for thirty-five years, and it's a comfort to have him across the table. We discuss problems that arise during the course of our surgeries, and many times two minds are better than one. We've been scrubbing our hands and forearms for ten minutes with an antiseptic soap. We dry our hands and arms with a sterile towel, and then we're gowned with light-green, paper gowns, which wrap around our entire bodies and tie in front. All the towels and drapes, which are simply large paper sheets, come from a surgical supply house and are already sterilized and wrapped individually in sterile outer packages. Every effort is made to keep contamination out of the room. Because we're so careful, the number of wound infections and complications from surgery is minimal.

The Operation

I now open Jim's abdomen and examine its entire contents, making mental notes of my findings. I not only want to check the extent of Jim's colon problem but also make sure he has no other abnormalities. I give special attention to Jim's liver, because colon cancer often spreads to the liver. In Jim's case that organ is free of metastasis, or spread. Next I examine the regional lymph nodes and notice that one is enlarged. I remove it and send it to the pathologist for a frozen section.

Ten minutes later, the pathologist's report is in. Jim's cancer seems pretty well contained in the colon, except for that lymph node, which contains cancer cells. We now know we have to be more radical in our resection (surgery to insure removal of all known cancer cells). I remove about eighteen inches of colon, from the mid portion of the transverse colon to a point about six inches above the anal outlet. This is what we call an *en bloc dissection*. I remove not only the bowel but also the *mesentery,* which is the apron that extends from the back wall of the abdomen to the bowel. Within the mesentery are blood vessels, lymph channels, and lymph nodes that are all encased in layers of fat. I don't want to handle the cancer too vigorously and dislodge cancer cells into blood vessels that could carry the cells to distant places in the body. Therefore, I isolate the large veins and tie them off, trapping any cancer cells and preventing them from floating.

The limits of the resection of Jim's tumor are now outlined in my mind. I make sure I cut well above and below the diseased area. It's better to take out too much rather than too little. Cancer is a killer, and if I take too little, islands of cancer cells may be left behind.

The outline of Jim's resection is V-shaped. The area includes some huge arteries, namely the left colic (one of the three arteries supplying the colon), which I isolate and tie with heavy sutures (stitches) to control bleeding. Sometimes the distortion of a tumor can lead into a trap, but the two surgeons can usually find a way out. As you might suspect, fat people are difficult to operate on because the mesentery, or fat apron in which the blood vessels are located, can be very thick, and the vessels can be very difficult to catch up with, especially if they are bleeding. In Jim's case, things go well, and the bloc resection goes according to plan.

We remove the colon section, with the mesentery, and send them to the pathologist for intensive examination. We approximate the borders of the mesentery with sutures, and we suture the two ends of the bowel together, much as you would splice two ends of a hose together. In Jim's case we do not need to do even a temporary colostomy (an opening in the bowel to prevent pressure on the stitches. This is closed in a few weeks—a very simple procedure).

We search Jim's abdomen for any bleeding points and take a sponge count. Each sponge we used must be accounted for. The sponges are counted before surgery; the small ones are put up in packets of twelve, which are counted by two people to verify the number before the sponges are dispensed. Then as they are used, they are laid out one by one on a paper on the floor. The circulating nurse announces whether or not the sponge count is correct. If it isn't, all progress is stopped until the missing sponge is located, even if it means taking an X ray on the operating table to make sure the sponge isn't hiding somewhere in the abdomen (each sponge has been marked with a substance the X ray will find).

Once the sponge count is verified, we close Jim's abdomen, apply dressings, and continue to control the anesthesia. Jim is placed on another gurney and is transported to the recovery room, where a staff of specially trained nurses will monitor and care for Jim as he awakens. Jim's operation has been a success.

After the Operation

While Jim has been in the operating room, his family has been pacing in the waiting room. Jim's operation took about two and a half hours. I follow Jim to the recovery room to make sure he's okay, write up his post-operative orders, and then go to the waiting room. I tell Jim's wife and two sons just how things went. The good thing was that we were able to get the tumor out without any compromise. The liver was free of involvement, and the resection went well. I can say that

I expect a full recovery, with an excellent prognosis to return to full activity. The only reservation I have is that one positive lymph node. That means we have to keep a close eye on Jim.

Our goal now is to get Jim over the effects of the surgery and get him out of the hospital. By that time we'll have a total report from the pathologist, who will dissect the specimen and search for more nodes in the mesentery. He'll also get a good look at the cell types, which will help further pinpoint the kind of tumor Jim had and the kind of further treatment he'll need.

My first post-op visit to Jim takes place that evening or early the next morning. Jim still feels groggy. But the nurses have made him take some deep breaths and hang his feet over the edge of the bed. Keeping his body a bit active keeps Jim from developing complications like clots in the calves of his legs, with the risk then of pulmonary embolus (a portion of clot breaking away and floating to the lungs, blocking an artery—can be very serious) or like a partial collapse of a portion of the lung. Jim is a little testy, which I see as a good sign.

I tell Jim during this visit that we got all the cancer and everything looks good. I haven't lied to Jim. But I haven't told him everything just yet. I have told Jim's wife what I will eventually tell him.

Pointing Toward Home

Right now Jim is getting only sips of water; his nutrition and electrolytes such as sodium, potassium, chloride, and calcium are being supplied through the IV. But already I've emphasized the goal of going home. Each day he takes a big step in that direction.

While Jim gathers his strength, we listen daily for evidence of bowel tones, a positive evidence that bowel function is returning. Now Jim can be given sips of clear liquid, like apple or cranberry juice. Gingerale and 7-Up are on Jim's list for early the next day.

When Jim is first able to pass gas, everyone gets excited. That is "the event," and now it's all downhill from here!

By this time Jim is out of bed and walking down the hall. If he has had enough antibiotics, his IV can be removed, along with his catheter. Jim is now on his own. And tomorrow, he's going home.

After Jim's stitches are taken out, he and I have a talk. I want to make it clear just where Jim is today and what his future holds. Jim now knows about the extension of the disease into the lymph nodes. As a matter of fact, the final report from the pathologist is in: Jim's cancer was an adenocarcinoma of the sigmoid colon, and he also has another cancerous lymph node in the mesentery. I now introduce Jim to the oncologist, who presents some options for Jim to think about.

Since Jim's type of cancer is not a good responder to any type of treatment other than surgery, he has four choices: radiation, chemotherapy, radiation and chemotherapy, or no further treatment. This is a very difficult decision to make because the statistics are so varied concerning the advantages of further treatment. This is where the art of medicine comes in. Jim is told that carcinoma of any portion of the gastrointestinal tract, from the mouth to the anus, is a resistant type of cancer and generally doesn't respond to radiation or chemotherapy. However, evidence suggests that radiation does kill young colon cancer cells, and every person's body is different. So the oncologist recommends radiation.

I tell Jim that I had cancer in the same location as his and that I chose radiation and chemotherapy, but I don't strongly recommend it for him. Why? My cancer was located at the same level as Jim's, but it arose from a different layer of the bowel. Mine came from a lymph node (a lymphoma). Jim's arose from the lining of the bowel, a glandular cell, and is an entirely different type of cancer. My tumor cells were highly susceptible to radiation and chemotherapy, while Jim's are very resistant. That's why each tumor has its own personality and must be treated in its own way.

Follow Up

The next week Jim visits me in my office. Jim has kept a journal for me on how he feels and anything that has happened. I examine his wound, check his blood for anemia, and record his weight. I increase his diet too. Of course, Jim wants to know what his chances are of full recovery. I tell him about a friend of mine who had a very similar cancer twenty-five years ago and has not had any evidence of a recurrence. It's time to dwell on the positive. Jim has at least a fifty-fifty chance of no recurrence. And even if the cancer does recur, further treatment is available. After thinking things over, Jim decides to take the advice of the oncologist and prepare for a course of radiation.

Two years later, Jim looks good. He's had no indication of recurrence. His weight is good. He feels good.

What did Jim learn through this experience? His priorities are different now. He watches his diet, exercises, and avoids anything that carries a known cancer risk. And Jim has experienced another change; he has learned to view each day of life as a gift and to accept that gift with thankfulness and hope.

QUESTIONS FOR THOUGHT
OR GROUP DISCUSSION

1. What are the advantages of surgical removal of cancer when this is possible?
2. What can I expect will happen to me or my loved one when going into the hospital for surgery?
3. Make a list of the steps described in this chapter. As you do, jot down any questions you would like to ask your doctor before any surgery takes place.
4. What ideas in this chapter help you feel confident that modern surgery is safe and effective?

4

WHAT TO EXPECT FROM RADIATION THERAPY

Of the three cancer treatments—surgery, radiation, and chemotherapy—I dreaded radiation the most. When my doctor told me I needed a course of radiation after my surgery, I felt really depressed. I had seen many people become ill under radiation treatment, so I began this phase of my treatment with a bias.

Still, I went daily for my rendezvous with the "cobalt bomb," fully expecting to become violently ill. But I never did. I had a total abdomen exposure, and I had been warned that radiation of the liver was very toxic. But I drove myself to my daily treatments and felt fine.

That's how it is in treating cancer. Everyone is different. In fact, my experience with radiation was actually pleasant. The radiologist was a great guy and always had a joke to brighten up the day. His two technicians were both fun people, who made an otherwise dull experience pleasant. After the first two weeks the technicians realized they could tease me, and tease me they did. If no one was in the waiting room when I came in, they would immediately say to me, "Take your pants down."

After about a week of that, I would enter with my belt unbuckled and say, "All right, I'm taking my pants down." And the last day I said, "Okay, I'm taking my pants down— for the last time!"

But I don't want to mislead you. Some people become very ill with radiation treatments. They experience nausea or have vomiting spells. And some feel exhausted and drained most of the time. More than one person has been tempted to give up in the middle of a course of radiation treatments, just because it made them feel so sick.

If radiation treatment makes you feel deathly ill, you're going to question whether or not you should continue with the treatments. You may wonder what good radiation therapy is doing for your body.

WHAT RADIATION THERAPY DOES

The goal of all cancer treatment is to destroy the cancer cells that infect your body. Radiation therapy uses controlled and powerful doses of high-energy radiation to kill cancer cells in your body. Radiation can have uncomfortable side effects, but we simply *have* to kill the cancer cells in your body. If we don't, the chances are terribly high that those cancer cells will kill you!

Very often, as in my case, all three treatment modes— surgery, radiation, and chemotherapy—were recommended. I didn't look forward to any of them with delight. But now, some fourteen years after my bout with cancer, I can tell you with certainty that it was sure worth any discomfort I experienced! These last years have been some of the richest of my life, and I wouldn't have missed them for anything.

If I had refused the treatments my doctors prescribed, I believe I *would* have missed them. Cancer would have killed me long ago.

Today radiation therapy is called by many different names—radiotherapy, X-ray therapy, cobalt therapy, X-ray treatments, irradiation, and radiation, to name a few. Whatever the name, radiation therapy directs high-intensity, invisible rays that damage the body's cells. These rays kill cancer cells that are *radiosensitive* (sensitive to the effects of radiation). Cells of the kidneys, testicles, and ovaries are carefully protected by lead shields when radiation therapy is given. Even cancers that are not especially sensitive to radiation are affected and tend to grow more slowly. So radiation is a powerful weapon against cancer—a weapon whose capabilities are constantly being sharpened and made even more effective.

Cancer treatment uses several different kinds of radiation. The source of the rays may be radioactive material (such as cobalt 60) or machines that generate X rays, gamma rays, neutron beams, beta rays, or electron beams. These rays may be directed at your cancer from outside, or a radiation source may be implanted directly in your body with a radioactive needle, for example. Sometimes radioactive elements are introduced by pill or intravenous injections.

Perhaps most important, today's computer-driven radiation machines are able to focus the radiation carefully on the target so that the maximum amount of rays are directed against the cancer itself and minimal damage is done to normal tissue. And our present, powerful cancer-conquering tools are soon to be supplemented by more potent successors. In 1991, after almost twenty years of work, Loma Linda University Medical

Center, in cooperation with Fermi National Accelerator Laboratory and the Proton Therapy Cooperative Group, will open the world's first hospital-based, patient-dedicated, proton-beam accelerator for the treatment of cancer. This type of X ray has been available in areas throughout the world for industrial use. Now it will be used in Loma Linda just for cancer patients. This beam will strike the target and the target only, without touching any other tissue. The $40-million facility is awesome. The equipment, including the accelerator and the guidance system, weighs 400 tons and produces up to 250 million electron volts of radiation.

The proton beam will significantly decrease injury to the healthy tissues it passes through. In contrast to conventional radiation, protons enter the body at a very low absorption rate and go through good tissues rapidly. Their energy deposition increases sharply at a specific point, called the Bragg Peak, where they release most of their energy. By focusing the Bragg Peak on a patient's tumor, most of the radiation is released at the site of the tumor, and damage to other tissues is significantly reduced. Proton-radiation treatments already performed by research machines have demonstrated startling results in the treatment of ocular melanoma, an almost always fatal cancer of the eye. Using the old atom smasher at the Harvard Cyclotron Laboratory, scientists have been able to eliminate the cancer in more than ninety-five percent of the cases and in most cases have been able to save the vision in the eye! The Loma Linda machine, with increased power, will be able to do what current machines can't do: reach deep cancers.

Your radiation treatments will be designed and supervised by a highly trained radiologist or radiation oncologist, who has a wide range of experience and radiation tools to use in treating your kind of cancer. Every step of your treatment will be designed just for you. The effect of the treatment on your cancer will be monitored, and the radiologist will adjust your course of treatment in view of your reaction to it. Even if you should have negative side effects, don't quit! Modern radiation treatments can kill many cancer cells—and save your life!

WALKING THROUGH RADIATION TREATMENTS

Radiation treatments are typically recommended instead of surgery in one of three situations: first, when the tumor can best be destroyed by radiation; second, when the tumor can be destroyed as effectively by radiation as by surgery; third, when the tumor can't be reached by surgery without destroying vital tissues. Radiation is the best treatment for some cancers, such as Hodgkin's disease and tumors in the lymph system. Frequently radiation is recommended along with other treatments.

To get a feel for what is likely to happen when you have your radiation therapy, let's follow Carol through her treatments.

Planning the Radiation Treatments

When Carol's primary-care physician recommended radiation treatments, she introduced Carol to a competent radiologist who lived in the next town and saw patients in the local hospital. (In some places this doctor might be called a radiology oncologist, radiation therapist, radiation oncologist, or therapeutic radiologist; whatever the name, the person is a medical doctor with special training in radiation therapy.)

Carol meets with her radiologist three times before starting treatment. During these visits her radiologist takes a careful history. He reviews all her records, including the pathology report that graded and staged her cancer. In Carol's case, he also orders a CT scan to define more clearly the exact site of her tumor. During this planning stage Carol's radiologist makes a number of complex computations to determine the dose and the timing of her treatments. It is comforting to Carol to realize that radiation treatments are designed specifically for her and that her doctor carefully considers every factor, from the grade and stage of her tumor, its location, whether it has spread, how her cancer type responds to radiation, her physical condition, and many other factors.

With the planning complete, her radiologist carefully explains the course of treatment he recommends. In Carol's case, the radiologist schedules twenty-five treatments: five weeks, at five days a week. He explains that if the total dose of radiation is given all at once, many of her normal cells would be killed along with the cancer cells. By dividing the dose needed to kill the cancer cells into a number of treatment doses, the healthy cells will have a chance to recuperate between treatments.

Carol asks about side effects, and the radiologist explains some of the possible reactions (see chart for some general and specific side effects). But she knows this is a life-or-death issue. She understands the reasons for the five-week series suggested and decides to go ahead.

At this point Carol's doctor carefully locates and marks on her body with indelible ink the *treatment port,* the area where the radiation is to be aimed. The mark will make sure the radiation can be directed at the same spot each treatment.

The Radiation Treatments

Carol's treatments are given at a nearby hospital's outpatient clinic. For the first three weeks, Carol drives herself to the daily appointments. She spends about an hour at the hospital, but only about thirty seconds under an X-ray machine. She quickly gets used to the routine.

When Carol comes for her treatment, she removes her clothes and puts on a hospital gown. The technician helps her get into position on the treatment table. The first time, Carol worries about pain, but she soon discovers the treatment involves no pain at all. Once or twice her legs cramp up because she has to lie totally still during the treatment, but that is all.

The technician puts lead shielding over parts of Carol's body that are not to be exposed and carefully positions the large machine over her body. When everything is exactly right, the technician leaves the room.

This is the worst moment for Carol. The big, heavy door closes, and she is alone. She feels slightly chilled on the cold table. The radiation machine hangs over her, and when it starts, she hears a hum that becomes faster and louder, like a jet-airplane engine. A trap window opens, and Carol knows rays are driving into her body. But the sense of panic lasts only for a moment. She knows those rays are killing her cancer. She knows that although she feels alone, she is carefully monitored over closed-circuit television. Best of all, it doesn't hurt and it only lasts for thirty seconds to a minute. She decides this is better than staying in the hospital.

If Carol's cancer had required an implant, using a needle or capsule to place radioactive material inside her body near the cancer site, Carol would need to be admitted to the hospital for two to six days. While she might not have experienced much discomfort, she would have needed to be in an isolated room, with few visitors. But, like most cancer patients, Carol didn't need an implant. In fact, radioactive implants (radium seeds) are being used less and less. So it is a relief each day, when the brief radiation treatment is over, to get into her own clothes and drive back to her home.

Three Weeks into Treatment

Carol doesn't feel sick during the first weeks of treatment. But halfway into the treatment time, she begins to experience some side effects. The worst, for her, is that she feels tired all the time. Carol is an active person who enjoys keeping busy. It is frustrating for her to feel so exhausted that she can hardly wait to get home from treatments to drop into bed. She feels guilty too. She can't even get her housework done, much less keep up with her part-time job.

Naturally Carol tells her diagnostic radiologist about her symptoms. First he explains that her symptoms are a natural reaction to radiation. Carol's body was telling her she needed more rest. The doctor suggests that she sleep when she feels tired and not force herself to do things she doesn't feel up to tackling. A daily nap and cutting down on visitors helps. It helps too when Carol is assured that the fatigue and other symptoms are temporary and will probably pass once her course of treatment is complete. If Carol had had a different reaction to her radiation treatment, her doctor might have given her the advice shown in the "Coping with Side Effects of Radiation Treatment" chart.

Carol and the doctor talk over the possibility of changing the treatment pattern to reduce the amount of radiation she receives weekly. But tests show her white-blood-cell count and platelet count are holding up, and Carol feels she would rather live with the side effects and get her treatment over rather than stretch them out.

One thing is especially encouraging. At the end of the third week the doctor takes a diagnostic X ray, which shows Carol that her tumor is actually shrinking. That buoys her up, even

COPING WITH SIDE EFFECTS
OF RADIATION TREATMENT

General Side Effects

Fatigue

Many people are able to work regular hours while taking radiation treatments. If you feel fatigued, get extra sleep and schedule daily rest periods. Your energy level will return to normal shortly after treatments end.

No appetite

Loss of appetite accompanied by nausea is frequently associated with radiation to the abdomen. Try tempting yourself with nutritious snacks, such as fruits, yogurt, and cottage cheese. Try new foods. Allure yourself with trips to new or unusual restaurants. This too will pass, but you need to eat to keep up your strength. Eating something light before and after treatments will help.

Sensitive skin

While skin burns are unusual, radiation often affects the layers just below the skin, making the skin sore or sensitive. Avoid strong soaps, perfumed lotions, cosmetics, direct sunlight, heating pads, or hot water bottles. If you are outdoors, apply sunblock. Cornstarch may be soothing.

Hair loss

Any hair in the direct path of the radiation can be affected. Typically the hair follicles are not destroyed but only injured. Hair will usually grow back after the treatment ends.

Specific Side Effects

Depending on where the radiation treatments are directed, side effects may include sore throat, vomiting, diarrhea, and other more rare reactions. Report your symptoms to your radiologist, who will offer suggestions or prescribe medicine.

though the last two weeks she didn't feel able to drive herself and had to rely on a friend to take her to her treatments.

Six Weeks After Radiation Treatments

Carol feels healthy again. Her energy has returned to normal, and the slight depression she had felt the last couple of weeks is gone.

Carol undergoes more diagnostic tests to help her radiologist evaluate the effectiveness of her course of treatments. In Carol's case, the tumor has been reduced, but it is still there. Her team of doctors consult and meet with her to talk about the future. Although Carol knows her fight with cancer isn't over yet, she feels encouraged. The radiation treatments have pushed the cancer back. She is confident that whatever comes next—more radiation or surgery or chemotherapy—she has hope for conquering her cancer.

And she is ready to take the next step.

QUESTIONS FOR THOUGHT OR GROUP DISCUSSION

1. What have you heard, read about, or experienced of side effects from radiation therapy?
2. Based on the "Coping with Side Effects of Radiation Treatment," what questions might you ask the radiologist about reducing side effects or discomfort?
3. What are the best reasons you can think of to take a course of radiation therapy despite possible unpleasant side effects?

5

WHAT TO EXPECT FROM CHEMOTHERAPY

Chemotherapy, which literally means "chemical therapy," is the third major resource in the fight against cancer. Many myths have developed about the use of drugs to treat cancer. Some people have the notion that chemotherapy is prescribed only as a last resort, when a case is hopeless. Others assume that the drugs aren't doing any good unless a person is really sick from side effects. Neither of these myths is true. What *is* true is that the medical community now has a powerful array of drugs that either kill cancer cells directly or interfere with their ability to grow and multiply.

Remember, the goal of your fight against cancer is to kill the cancer cells that have begun to multiply in your body. Some cancers can be treated by surgery and/or radiation, powerful doses of high-intensity energy focused on the tumor. Still other cancers are best treated by chemicals that are toxic to various cancer cells. The National Cancer Institute estimates that fifteen percent of cancers can be conquered by chemotherapy alone. Used in conjunction with other treatments, the effectiveness of chemotherapy is multiplied. Doctors may prescribe all three modes of treatment for a single case.

But chemotherapy has an important drawback—side effects.

SIDE EFFECTS OF CHEMOTHERAPY

Soon after my own experience with chemotherapy, I was attending a medical society cancer seminar in San Diego. As Dr. Vincent DiVita of the National Cancer Institute discussed the various agents that could be used to battle a particular cancer, he mentioned two drugs that had given me a lot of trouble.

I cornered Dr. DiVita after the meeting and, half kidding, accused him of throwing poison around with total disregard for how it was going to make the patient feel. He freely admitted that the side effects of the various drugs were all too often ignored in the enthusiasm for their destructive effect on the cancer. After all, he said, the important thing was saving a patient's life!

We had a very constructive discussion, and I hope I impressed him that the oncologist must never forget that on the other end of those poisonous chemicals are sensitive human beings who must live with their side effects. If the side effects are too unbearable, the patient may opt to discontinue the entire treatment program. I've seen it happen too often.

Now, believe me, I can empathize. I wasn't adversely affected by my radiation treatments. But my chemotherapy was something else! I don't appreciate at all the oncologist who says, "There's nothing to it," or, "Oh, it may make you a little nauseous and dizzy." Personally, I would much rather prepare for the worst. If I find out I'm one of the many who find the side effects are bearable, then I'm pleasantly surprised. On the other hand, if the side effects are worse than I'm expecting, I can easily become depressed, making the treatments even harder to bear.

Let me help you understand what the chemotherapy experience is like by describing my own treatments. As I do, remember I took my course of treatments in 1977—*and I've been free of cancer ever since!* I wouldn't want to go through chemotherapy again, but I'm truly glad I hung in there, despite the side effects that made me so sick.

My first bothersome side effect was nausea and vomiting. Now, I'm not an easy vomiter. I make a big production out of it as I drape myself over the toilet bowl. Chemotherapy made me so sick that at times I wished I could die rather than vomit anymore. The trouble is, when I wasn't vomiting, I felt as if I was going to. The chemical that did this to me was vincristine, which I took intravenously every three weeks. For about a week afterward I would keep on throwing up, and during that time I was a real dog to live with. My wife, Genevieve, was terrific, encouraging me and waiting on me during my down times. I didn't want visitors around then, just one person. That was no time for company and no time for small talk. In fact, small talk made me crazy. I'm sure I insulted more than one person during these times. My appetite went to zero, and Genevieve kept trying to get food down me, enriched with vitamins, protein—anything to build up my body. I took antinausea medication. But if it was working, I hate to think what condition I would have been in without it!

Then I also took a high dosage of prednisone, and that altered my psyche. I felt very strange. I had dreams, ares really, that made no sense. When I woke up, I was agitated and hyper. My reasoning was altered. I felt numbness and tingling in my extremities. I'm a rather easygoing person, but I became easily irritated and hostile under the influence of chemotherapy. To top it off, I also had cramps and diarrhea. Then I lost my hair. All of it. I can almost guarantee that when you have chemotherapy, you'll lose your hair too. Of course, when my treatments were over, my hair came back in again. In fact, it came back in thicker than before, and all the grey was gone—well, for a while. Many people buy wigs to use during their bald period. I wore a Greek fisherman's cap, which led to one of those comical incidents that helps lighten up even our most painful times. One morning as I was leaving the hospital, I ran across a drunk commercial fisherman who had had a bad night. He was sitting at the entrance waiting for a ride, and when he saw me in my cap, he sat up and hollered, "Taxi!" That made my day and has given me many a laugh since. You need those times of comic relief during your treatment.

But the greatest relief came when my doctor told me I had had enough. After six months of chemotherapy, I could have kissed my oncologist when he told me!

The months that I spent on chemotherapy were, quite honestly, terrible. But the years of healthy, cancer-free life that those months helped purchase made them totally worthwhile. I would go through it all over again, gladly. Chemotherapy hurts. But it pays tremendous dividends down the road.

HOW CHEMOTHERAPY WORKS

The use of chemotherapy in the fight against cancer dates back to World War II, when researchers were studying the effect of poisonous gases on human tissue. They learned that mustard gas had a toxic affect on actively multiplying tissues—which is just what cancer is: tissues that multiply wildly. Yale researchers found that nitrogen mustard gas could be used to attack cancers of the lymph system and bone marrow.

During the 1960s and 1970s, the use of chemicals in the fight against cancer expanded rapidly. Many new chemicals were tested and found effective against selected cancers. Researchers learned that cells go through a series of stages in the process of multiplying. Some drugs attack the cancer at particular stages of its life cycle, while others attack it continuously. By using combinations of drugs and carefully timing their administration, today's doctors mount sophisticated, effective assaults on many tumors.

Doctors often repeat courses of chemotherapy because analysis has shown that the rate of destruction of malignant cells is a function of "first order kinetics." That is, the process of killing cancer cells proceeds at a relatively constant level: if seventy-five percent of a tumor's cells are killed by one dose of a drug, a second dose will kill seventy-five percent of the remaining twenty-five percent. By giving repeated courses, the number of cancer cells can often be reduced to a level that the body's own immune system can handle.

Another reason why chemotherapy is given in intermittent courses of treatment is that cancer-fighting chemicals are powerful poisons—poisons that affect healthy cells as well. Some of these poisons drastically suppress the immune system's natural ability to fight not only cancer but also other illnesses. If the immune system is given seven to fourteen days to recover between treatments, the body maintains better health during the cancer battle.

Despite the drawback of uncomfortable side effects, chemotherapy offers several positive dynamics in the cancer-recovery process. First, chemotherapy has one unique advantage over surgery and radiation. Surgery and radiation can affect a cancerous mass, but they can't touch smaller colonies of cancer cells that may have drifted into other parts of the body through the blood or lymph systems. But chemicals injected or absorbed through the stomach can travel through the bloodstream to wherever cancer cells may grow!

Second, chemotherapy can enhance both surgery and radiation: chemotherapy shrinks tumors so that they can be removed by surgery, and chemotherapy makes radiation treatments more effective. Third, chemotherapy alone can kill some forms of cancer, and it can achieve long-term remission in other forms of cancer. By itself or in combination with other standard medical treatments, chemotherapy gives us a terrific edge in our effort to conquer cancer!

CHEMICAL AGENTS

Not long ago I received the June 1989 *Medical Letter on Drugs and Therapeutics,* which listed forty-one commercially available cancer-treatment drugs used in the United States and Canada and thirteen other cancer-fighting drugs used in tests run by the National Cancer Institute. Each of these drugs is a powerful tool in the fight against cancer, especially when used in combination with other drugs.

In the "Chemotherapy" chart, I've described a number of drugs that fight specific cancers, along with any major side effects the drugs have on most people. People are different and respond differently to drug therapy, so you may have additional or different side effects from any of these. But it may help you to be prepared when a particular drug is known to create certain side effects.

But my main reason for giving you this list isn't to warn

you about side effects; it's to give you a sense ᵥ confidence. It's to remind you that today's doctors ᵢ large arsenal of chemical weapons to help you win your battlᵥ with cancer. The point I'm trying to make is that just as the medical community has made tremendous advances in surgery and radiation treatment, they've also made great progress in the kinds of chemotherapy that will give you a significant edge in your fight against cancer. Yes, new medical miracles do loom just over the horizon. But the range of chemical agents that effectively battle cancer *now* would have seemed like a medical miracle thirty, twenty, or even ten years ago.

CHEMOTHERAPY

Data Chart

Drugs & Hormones*	Cancers treated	Possible side effects
Adrenocorticoids*	Hodgkin's disease, lukemias, lymphomas, breast, myelomas	appetite increase, fluid retention, mood swings, rash, weight gain, ulcers, weakness, high blood sugar
Androgens*	breast	nausea, vomiting, fluid retention, weight gain, liver toxicity, hair growth, irregular menstruation, voice lowered
Antiestrogens*	breast	brief nausea, vomiting, hot flashes, vaginal discharge, itching, headache, light-headedness
Asparaginase (Elspar)	leukemia	nausea, vomiting, allergic skin and pulmonary reactions,

Drugs & Hormones*	Cancers treated	Possible side effects
		lowered blood count, lethargy, depression
Bleomycin (Blenoxane)	cervix, testicle, lymphomas, squamous cell carcinomas, skin	skin rash, hair loss, mouth sores, fever, chills, weight loss, vomiting, allergic reactions, loss of appetite
Busulfan (Myleran)	chronic myelogenous leukemias	tiredness, lowered blood count, enlarged male breasts, nausea, weight loss, skin and pulmonary reactions
Carmustine	colon, melanomas, brain, stomach, pancreas, lung, liver, myelomas, lymphomas	nausea, vomiting, liver, lung pain, lowered blood count
Chlorambucil (Leukeran)	breast, ovary, testicle, lymphomas, leukemia (lymphocytic)	nausea, lowered blood count
Cisplatin (Platinol)	ovary, testicle, lung, head and neck, prostate, cervix, bladder, osteogenic sarcoma	severe nausea, vomiting, dulled hearing, loss of feeling in arms and legs, lowered blood count, joint pain, kidney damage
Cyclophosphamide (Cytoxan and Neosar)	breast, lung, ovary, cervix, lymphomas, leukemias, myelomas, neuroblastoma, sarcomas	nausea, vomiting, problem with fluids, lowered blood count, bladder infection
Cytarabine (Cytosar-U)	leukemias, lymphomas	lowered blood count, nausea, vomiting

WHAT TO EXPECT FROM CHEMOTHERAPY

Drugs & Hormones*	Cancers treated	Possible side effects
Dacarbazine (DTIC-Dome)	Hodgkin's disease, melanoma, sarcomas	nausea, vomiting, fever, weakness, lowered blood count, loss of appetite
Dactinomycin (Cosmegen)	testicle, uterus, choriocarcinoma, sarcomas, Wilms' tumor, rhabdomyosarcoma	nausea, vomiting, diarrhea, hair loss, mouth sores, skin eruptions, lowered blood count
Daunorubicin (Cerubidine)	acute leukemias	nausea, vomiting, red urine, fever, hair loss, lowered blood counts, heart problems
Doxorubicin (Adriamycin)	leukemias, lymphomas, lung, breast, liver, stomach, bladder, sarcomas, prostate, testicle, head and neck, thyroid, Wilms' tumor	vomiting, hair loss, red urine, mouth sores, lowered blood count, heart problems
Estramustine (Emcyt)	prostate	nausea, vomiting, diarrhea, enlarged male breast
Estrogens* (DES)	breast, prostate	nausea, vomiting, weight gain, swelling of breasts, headache, stopped menstruation, loss of calcium, bleeding
Etoposide (VePesid)	testicle, lung, lymphomas, leukemias	nausea, vomiting, constipation, hair loss, low blood count, loss of appetite, nerve disorders
Floxuridine (FUDR)	liver	nausea, vomiting, diarrhea, low blood

87

CONQUERING CANCER

Drugs & Hormones*	Cancers treated	Possible side effects
		count, mouth sores, loss of appetite
Flourouracil (Fluorouracil, Adrucil, Efudes)	breast, ovary, colon, rectum, stomach, cervix, skin, bladder, pancreas	nausea, vomiting, diarrhea, mouth sores, hair loss, lowered blood count
Hydroxyurea (Hydrea)	leukemia, head and neck, kidney, prostate, melanoma	nausea, vomiting, lowered blood count, constipation, mouth sores, diarrhea, rash
Lomustine (CeeNu)	brain, colon, lung, melanoma, Hodgkin's disease	nausea, vomiting, lowered blood count, hair loss, loss of appetite
Mechlorethamine (Mustargen)	Hodgkin's desease, lymphomas, lung	nausea, vomiting, hair loss, lowered blood count, metallic taste
Melphalan (Alkeran)	ovary, breast, testicle, melanoma, multiple myeloma	nausea, vomiting, diarrhea, lowered blood count, mouth sores, skin eruption
Mercaptopurine (Purinethol)	leukemias	nausea, vomiting, lowered blood count, loss of appetite
Methotrexate	breast, cervix, lung, head and neck, lymphomas, choriocarcinoma, various sarcomas	nausea; vomiting; diarrhea; mouth sores; liver, kidney and pulmonary problems; lowered blood count
Mitomycin (Mutamycin)	pancreas, colon, breast, lung, gastric	nausea, vomiting, lowered blood count, kidney problems
Mitotane (Lysodren)	adrenal	nausea, vomiting, diarrhea, loss of

WHAT TO EXPECT FROM CHEMOTHERAPY

Drugs & Hormones*	Cancers treated	Possible side effects
		appetite, rash, vision problems, confusion
Plicamycin (Mithracin)	testicle	nausea, vomiting, lowered blood count, loss of appetite, headaches, lethargy, skin rash, liver and kidney problems
Procarbazine (Matulane)	Hodgkin's disease, lymphomas, lung, brain	nausea, vomiting, lowered blood count, joint and muscle pain, depression, severe reaction to alcohol
Progesterones*	kidney, breast, prostate	mild stomach trouble, breast enlargement, tenderness
Streptozocin (Zanosar)	pancreas, Hodgkin's disease, carcinoid tumors	nausea, vomiting, lowered blood count, low blood sugar, headaches, weakness, kidney damage
Thioguanine	leukemias	lowered blood count
Thio-TEPA	breast, ovaries, bladder, Hodgkin's disease	loss of appetite, lowered blood count
Vinblastine (Velban)	lymphomas, testicle, breast, some carcinomas	hair loss, stomach pain, constipation, lowered blood count, vomiting, nerve disorders
√ Vincristine (Oncovin)	leukemias, lymphomas, Hodgkin's disease, breast, sarcomas, Wilms' tumor, neuroblastoma	constipation, hair loss, jaw and abdominal pain, nerve disorders

For more information on chemotherapy, write to the United States Department of Health and Human Services and ask for the helpful booklet entitled "Chemotherapy and You: A Guide to Self-Help During Treatment."

When I think back over my medical career and realize how far we've come from that mid-40s discovery that mustard gas was an anticancer agent, I can't help being amazed. And thankful too. How much more optimistic we can be today when someone is diagnosed with cancer. How thrilled I am to be able to offer you *honest* hope!

WALKING THROUGH
CHEMOTHERAPY TREATMENTS

Even though I've shared my own experience with chemotherapy, I want to walk you through Bill's experience with chemotherapy too. Bill has an abdominal tumor that has not been completely removed by surgery.

Bill's primary medical team is made up of his family doctor, a diagnostic radiologist, a surgeon, and a medical oncologist. Bill has had successful abdominal surgery, but the pathologist found evidence that some cancer cells had broken off and have settled into nearby lymph nodes. No one can tell how far the cancer has spread or where colonies of cancer cells might be breeding another life-threatening tumor. The team agrees that surgery should be followed up by chemotherapy.

Bill isn't particularly happy with the news, but as his doctor explains the situation, he realizes that starting chemotherapy soon after surgery is the safest course he can take.

Planning the Chemotherapy

Planning a course of chemotherapy, which calls for a thorough knowledge of the cancer drugs and how they affect various tumors, is the task of the team's medical oncologist. The oncologist considers a host of factors: which drugs to use, which dosage to prescribe, which method to introduce the drugs into the system, and so on. Once again Bill's medical records, pathology reports, and X rays are studied, and he is given yet another thorough physical. The oncologist also is interested in Bill's general attitude and notes Bill's strong will to be able to return to work.

After assembling all the relevant information available, the oncologist sets up a second appointment to discuss the course of chemotherapy she would recommend.

Bill has a lot of questions at that second meeting, particularly because he is uneasy about chemotherapy. He needs to get back to work as soon as possible because his sick leave is nearly used up. He doesn't think he can afford to miss much more time. How sick will he feel from the prescribed chemicals? Is it really worthwhile taking this route? Can the side effects be limited in some way? And what kinds of reactions to the therapy should he report to the doctor?

Bill's oncologist explains that she will start him on an "induction dose"—large amounts of the drug for the first few days, followed by smaller doses—allowing her to plan a sequence of drugs, timing the cycles so that the worst side effects would be on weekends rather than during the work week. The doctor does, however, emphasize several things.

First, she emphasizes that Bill must follow *exactly* the schedule for taking the drugs. Timing is vital because the different drugs prescribed are carefully sequenced to have maximum impact on the cancer.

Second, she goes over all other drugs Bill presently is taking to make sure they will produce no interaction with the cancer treatments.

Third, the oncologist reassures Bill about the side effects.

Not everyone has a strong reaction to the drugs. In most cases nausea and vomiting start a few hours after a treatment and last a short time. Some people feel sick for twelve hours or a day; others feel a persistent nausea.

Finally, she explains to Bill some possible but unusual side effects associated with each medication. The oncologist wants Bill to feel totally comfortable about calling her if any unusual, severe symptoms occur. She tells Bill to report any fever over 100°, bleeding or bruising, strong allergic reaction, shortness of breath, unusually intense pain, headaches, severe diarrhea, or bloody urine. Bill is a little frightened to realize some of the possible side effects of his chemotherapy. But he would rather know what to expect than be surprised by some strange symptoms. And it comforts Bill to know that he can call the oncologist at any time. After Bill and the oncologist talk, he feels comfortable enough to go ahead with the course of treatments.

Administering the Chemotherapy

Chemicals can be introduced into the body in a number of ways: some are delivered directly to a tumor by use of a catheter; some are injected into the vein; others are administered in pill form. In Bill's case, the oncologist uses two drugs at first: one is injected every fourth Friday afternoon and the other, a pill, is taken daily for three weeks, with a seven-day break after each three-week sequence. Bill finds that the first two days after the injection are really rough and that he feels sick the hour after taking his pill. He finds that if he takes his pill in the late afternoon, he can avoid feeling sick at work, but it makes it a little rough on the family when his nausea makes him irritable and depressed.

Monitoring the Chemotherapy

The chemicals used in chemotherapy are poisonous to the body, and their impact on general health has to be monitored carefully. One possible side effect is depression of the bone marrow, which means that the bone marrow's ability to make red and white blood cells is decreased.

As a result, Bill has frequent blood tests. Too few red cells will make it difficult for Bill's bloodstream to transport enough oxygen throughout his body and would cause tiredness or dizziness. Too few white cells will limit his body's ability to fight infection. If his blood count drops too low, Bill's doctor will order transfusions or will temporarily stop his chemotherapy. At one point, Bill's blood count drops, but the drop is not low enough to warrant transfusions or cessation of therapy; he is simply encouraged to keep on eating a healthy diet.

A second reason oncologists monitor chemotherapy is to see how the tumor is responding. In Bill's case, the oncologist couldn't measure the tumor because there was no specific site against which the cancer was localized. But generally, response can be measured in two ways: a *complete* response means that all observable evidence of the disease is gone, and a *partial* response means that a dramatic reduction of the measurable disease is achieved. By monitoring the tumor, an oncologist can tell when a particular course of treatment is ineffective and can switch to different combinations of drugs.

Change in Treatment

Bill's first course of chemotherapy is not intended to reduce a specific tumor but to kill invisible cancer cells that may have remained in his body after his surgery. In planning Bill's course of treatment, the oncologist makes some very educated guesses as to what chemicals, in which combination and sequences, would best do that job.

After three months of the first treatment course, the oncologist tells Bill it's time to introduce a different treatment—a four-month course of different drugs. The bad news is that Bill will lose his hair—not just the hair on his head, *all* his hair. The good news is that the new treatment is proven to be effective against his type of cancer. She assures Bill that his hair will grow back after the four-month course is over.

People prepare for hair loss in a variety of ways. Some just grin and bear it. Others buy a wig. The doctor suggests that if Bill wants to disguise his hair loss, he should buy a hairpiece before the treatments begin. That way he can match his hair color, and as the hair begins to thin, he can camouflage the transition. Many people consider this a good option. Some insurance companies cover the cost of wigs or hairpieces for cancer treatment, and the Internal Revenue Service treats them as a tax-deductible expense.

Bill hesitates a bit as he thinks about the new treatment course the oncologist proposes. But he decides that the temporary loss of his hair is a relatively small price to pay for an even better chance at recovery.

After Chemotherapy

At the end of Bill's seven months of chemotherapy, there is no way to pronounce him "cured." Instead, the doctor and Bill conclude that they have done everything possible to destroy any cancer cells that had remained in his body. Bill realizes that he will have to live with the possibility of recurrence for several years before he will know if the cancer is gone.

But the uncertainty doesn't weigh on Bill's mind as he once thought it would. Bill has learned the important lesson: The battle isn't easy, and there is no *absolute* guarantee that a person will survive, but the possibilities are very high that with the help of surgery, radiation, and chemotherapy, most people will conquer cancer.

And the chances of a cure are getting better all the time! The National Cancer Institute reports that every year, 50,000 substances are tested for their impact on cancer. And researchers constantly test new schedules and doses to make the effective drugs even more powerful. So even if your reaction to chemotherapy is as painful as mine was, don't quit. Life is a precious gift. It really is worth fighting to preserve.

QUESTIONS FOR THOUGHT
OR GROUP DISCUSSION

1. What have you heard, read about, or experienced of side effects from chemotherapy?
2. Based on the "Chemotherapy" chart, what questions might you ask the oncologist about reducing side effects or discomfort?
3. What are the best reasons you can think of to take a course of chemotherapy despite possible unpleasant side effects?
4. Consider: If chemotherapy makes you or your loved one sick, what do you suppose it is doing to your cancer?

6

TAKING CHARGE

Gloria was a beautiful thirty-two-year-old Eurasian woman with gorgeous skin and features. She came to me because she had noticed a growth in her breast. It was especially alarming to her because she made her living as a model.

When I saw Gloria, she was obviously anxious and upset. After I examined her, I explained we couldn't tell exactly what the growth was until we could do a biopsy (obtain and examine some of the tissues making up the growth). She wasn't sure she wanted the biopsy. Wouldn't that leave a scar on her breast? I assured her that it would be a tiny scar, that all we would do was take a little piece, find out what it was, and then go on from there. She said she would let me know.

In a couple of days she called back and said she was ready to talk. When Gloria and her husband came to my office, I wanted to explain to both of them as clearly as possible what Gloria's situation was. As I talked, I noticed that Gloria got more and more quiet. Her anxiety soon turned into pronounced withdrawal. I ended up talking to her husband, with Gloria listening in almost as a passive onlooker. I explained that if, when we did the biopsy, the results indicated she had cancer, we should go ahead and do the surgery at that time. I told them that surgery was important, even if it meant that part of her breast would need to be removed because her life was much more important than her job or anything else. When she heard that, she became extremely quiet. She didn't even ask any questions. Her husband asked a few questions and said they would get back to me.

In a couple of days they were back. They decided they would have only the biopsy done. She wanted to wake up from the surgery and then decide how much more she wanted done.

In the hospital, I did a real small incision on her breast, got a piece of tissue, and sent it down to the pathologist. It was cancer. When I told her husband, Ed, he shook his head and said, "This is going to be a real rough go because Gloria isn't going to want anything done."

When she awakened from the surgery, I told her what we had found. She said almost nothing. She just wanted to go home. I said she could go home, but I reminded her we weren't through yet. She hadn't been treated.

In a couple of days Gloria and her husband came back to my office. She was still very quiet. I told her exactly what she had to do—she needed more surgery. Then she did begin to ask some questions. "Is this going to cure me?" "Is this going to disfigure me?" "Do I have any chance of survival?" "Just what am I up against?"

I tried to paint as bright a picture as I could, but it was a bad situation. Reluctantly, she decided to have the surgery done. As we got ready for her surgery, I tried to prepare her psychologically. I told her there was real hope for her recovery and that we would worry about the modeling when we needed to. We could even do plastic surgery, if she wanted it.

When we began the surgery, we discovered that the cancer was much worse than it had appeared to be. Her lymph nodes were positive, and the cancer had spread through her breast into the muscle. We had to do a really radical mastectomy.

When she awakened and found out what had happened, she became even more quiet. Extremely quiet. She got to the point where she showed no expression, no facial motion at all. She became severely depressed.

I saw her many times after her surgery, ostensibly to change her dressings, but really to try to break through the depression and give her something or someone in whom she could place her trust. I described my own cancer and my own reactions. Though my reactions weren't as severe as hers, my case was enough like hers that she knew I understood. The most important thing I told her was that she needed to find something she could depend on, something that would give her support through this time.

I knew when I was talking with Gloria that she had a long, hard battle ahead. Nearly all cancer patients do. And while medical science provides many powerful weapons and skilled doctors use them effectively, a lot still depends on *what the cancer patient contributes*.

What worried me about Gloria was that her depression might lead her into lethargy and she would give up. We couldn't afford that. Gloria needed to become an active participant in her fight against cancer. I needed her full involvement on the team. She had a choice: She could choose to give up, or she could choose to become part of the fight against her cancer.

TAKING CHARGE

What is Gloria's part in her fight? What can any cancer patient do to facilitate his or her recovery?

Let me share with you some coping strategies, some good news about pain, and some straight talk about health habits and the role of mental attitude. Then I'll tell you what I shared with Gloria about the need for something to depend on, to support her through this difficult time.

COPING

Some people cope well with cancer; others do not. Someone may say, "I've got a little bit of cancer," accept treatment, and start planning vacation trips to take when the treatment is over. The confident expectation that everything will go well is one way of coping. Others may say, "I've got a really bad cancer" and get themselves ready for battle, keeping careful records of treatments, responses, setbacks, and progress. Active involvement that gives these people a sense of control is another way of coping. Either approach may work for you, though each has its drawbacks: The optimist may be devastated by a setback, and the fighter may become obsessed with the disease. But these are personal strategies. They may work for one person and not for another.

Many coping patterns work, and you'll probably develop one that suits your own personality. Whatever strategy you develop, it can do something very important for you. It can give you a sense of control, a feeling that you have a say in your own future.

Studies done on two groups of cancer patients—those who cope well and those who do not cope well—suggest that the people within these two groups have several common characteristics.

People who do not cope well:
- deny their illness, even refusing or stopping treatment.
- hold in their emotions and withdraw from others.
- continue to feel intense anger, which may turn inward as depression.
- blame themselves or others for their disease.
- refuse to talk with others about their feelings and refuse counseling help.
- burst out erratically against others.
- refuse intimacy with loved ones.
- wallow in self-pity and constantly ask, Why me?
- expect some magical cure, with or without treatment.
- give up.

People who do cope well:
- seek and rely on good medical care.
- gather information that will help them understand their condition but do not fixate on data that might make them feel anxious.
- share their apprehensions openly with family and friends.
- keep a balance between self-reliance and getting help when needed from counselors, family, and friends.
- remain hopeful, but don't kid themselves.
- are realistic about their limitations during treatment and do the things that are most important to them.
- accept responsibility for their diet, self-care, and plans for the future.
- keep working and maintain their normal routine as much as possible.
- set limited, attainable goals.
- get their mind off themselves.
- maintain religious faith.

TAKING CHARGE

As we look at these characteristics, perhaps the most important thing we see is that people who cope well assume they have an important role in their battle with cancer and that they have control over how they react to the disease. They are honest with themselves and others. They are realistic, and yet they maintain that important sense of hope.

Now, this doesn't mean you have to act like some superman or superwoman, to shrug off the threat of cancer and breeze through the months or even years of cancer treatment with nothing but a happy smile. You will have times of utter discouragement and depression—every cancer patient does. You will have times of wanting to give up. It's all right to have these feelings. But it's not all right to let them dominate you to the extent that you *do* give up.

It's all right to have times when you're short-tempered, envious, or bitter. We're all human, and such feelings wash over us at times. But it's not all right to drive your loved ones away rather than accept their support. It's not all right to let bitterness fester inside, racking you with self-pity and hostility toward others.

When those emotions come, and they will, you'll need to take charge—whether or not you feel like it. You'll need to check your coping patterns against the list of positive characteristics and make some changes if that's necessary.

The thing to remember is that you are not helpless. How you battle your cancer *does* matter. You play a vital role in conquering your cancer.

COPING WITH PAIN

One of cancer patients' greatest fears is pain. This is a realistic worry, in one sense. Many cancers are painful. Many cancer treatments are painful. The Harvard Medical School

Health Letter reports that between sixty and ninety percent of patients with life-threatening cancer will have pain intense enough to require narcotics. But that pain comes late in the game and can be dealt with when it occurs.

Pain was never a problem with my patients. They had pain, but I was able to help them manage it. I believe that if a patient has severe pain, it's the doctor's fault. I tried to stay ahead of my patients, anticipating the pain they would encounter and taking steps to minimize that pain before it became a problem for them. Today's medical advances can control pain to the extent that no cancer patient needs to be overcome by it.

This brings me to another of those important ways in which you can take responsibility for the treatment of your cancer. You can communicate your symptoms—including symptoms of pain—to your doctor. Part of the problem with pain is that its cause isn't always easy to diagnose. Your pain may be associated with expansion of a primary tumor. It may be linked to the spread of cancer. It may be caused by the treatment—surgery, chemotherapy, or radiation. It may not have any direct relationship to the cancer at all. Keeping the communication lines open with your doctor is really important. He or she will want to locate the source of your pain, not only because it will give important information about the progress of your treatment but also because then an effective pain treatment can be prescribed.

Pain can be treated a variety of ways today. First, the source of the pain can be attacked. If you have a tumor in a bone, radiation focused on that spot often will relieve the pain with no negative side effects. Some tumors that cause pain can be removed surgically or can be shrunk by chemotherapy.

Second, the transmission of localized pain can be blocked. Some drugs suppress pain signals so that the nerves do not carry the pain message to the brain, preventing you from feeling it. Or some people find relief through an injection of a local anesthetic.

Third, we can also block the *perception* of pain, so that even when pain signals reach the brain, they cause less distress. While some people have success with bio-feedback techniques, narcotic drugs are the most powerful resource here.

Your doctor will know how to treat both mild and intense pain and will help tailor a pain-control program that will meet your particular needs. As long as you communicate your needs to your doctor, you needn't be anxious about feeling the intense pain associated with some of the more serious cancers.

HEALTH HABITS

One of the most important things you can do to help yourself is to work toward a healthy lifestyle. That involves eating a balanced diet and maintaining your weight. It also calls for drinking plenty of fluids—fruit juices, carbonated soft drinks, and water—in order to keep your urine output high.

Regular exercise is also important, particularly recreational, outdoor exercise. Golf, tennis, swimming, and walking all make the heart and lungs work more effectively. Studies show that during exercise, our brains produce endorphins, proteins that act as natural pain killers. Keep active and push yourself to your level of tolerance, and then move just a bit beyond that.

As much as exercise is important, so is rest. If that means that you need to lie down during the day or take a nap, then make sure you do that.

Many books and magazines contain a lot of misinformation

about the role of diet in a cancer patient's life. A balanced diet is important because it helps you maintain your strength and rebuilds normal tissues that may be affected by your treatment. Eating well also helps you withstand the side effects of radiation and chemotherapy treatments. If you eat right, you'll have fewer infections and be less susceptible to other diseases. Diet can make a big difference.

But watch out. Be particularly skeptical when you read about miraculous healing achieved by special cancer diets. For instance, one fad diet, the "macrobiotic diet," has been adapted for cancer patients. This diet typically consists of about 60 percent whole grains, 25 percent vegetables, 15 percent beans and sea vegetables, and 5 percent soups. Now while that sounds perfectly healthy, the diet has two problems: First, macrobiotic diets often leave out vital nutrients (vitamins C and D, and iron) and typically are short on the calories that provide energy; second, the loudest proponents of macrobiotic diets label traditional cancer treatments "violent," "toxic," and "unnatural." Many actually urge cancer patients to abandon "harmful" radiation or chemotherapy treatments—the very treatments that can save your life! Other people turn to off-beat cures, the most common of which rely on a "metabolic therapy" that combines a special diet with colon cleansing, vitamins, minerals, and enzymes. It's easy to understand why some people turn to these treatments that promise cures based on a "more natural" way to eat.

What may surprise you is that educated people are most vulnerable to the lure of non-conventional therapies. These people don't passively follow the doctor's orders but read and search for information about their disease. Since you're reading this book, it means you may well be in that group of vulnerable people! Because your cancer treatment may call for a long-term commitment to uncomfortable courses of chemotherapy or radiation, you'll probably be tempted to grasp hold of some of the unproven claims and theories. They may very well look like a reasonable way out. A University of Pennsylvania Cancer Center study showed sixty percent of those people using unorthodox cancer treatments were doing it in conjunction with their doctor's treatment (most without telling their doctor they were involved in other treatments besides the therapy he or she had prescribed). But the other forty percent of those relying on unorthodox treatments had stopped seeing their doctor altogether!

But be very careful. Before you turn to these non-conventional treatments, talk with your doctor. If you're feeling sick from the side effects of your therapy or discouraged because your cancer has been slow to respond, talk with your doctor. He or she knows good options for you and will help you get through the hard times.

If you still wish to try an enthusiastically promoted cancer-curing diet, *please* tell your doctor. He or she may not like it. Your doctor will know that the American Cancer Society has concluded that macrobiotic diets provide *no* benefits to cancer patients. In fact, the American Cancer Society warns against such diets. But your doctor must be informed about what you're doing. First, your doctor has to make sure that nothing you're doing interacts negatively with the treatments he or she has ordered. Second, your doctor needs to know if your diet lacks any essential dietary elements.

Most important of all, don't abandon medically proven treatments for unproven theories and practices, no matter how enthusiastic the testimonies of those who have been "cured." Diet *can* help you in your fight against cancer. But it has to be a healthy diet, a balanced diet that supplies all your nutritional needs. Your doctor will introduce you to the staff nutritionist, who will tailor your diet to your individual needs. He or she will be available to consult with you at any time during the course of your treatment.

PREVENTION

We are all interested in preventing cancer if at all possible. More causes for cancer are being uncovered all the time, and those causes help dictate our lifestyle. Here are some general rules to follow which will help you avoid cancer.

What Are the Protective Factors?

1. Eat more cabbage-family vegetables. These vegetables appear to protect you against colorectal, stomach, and respiratory cancers. They include broccoli, brussels sprouts, all cabbages, and kale.

2. Add more high-fiber foods. A high-fiber diet may protect you against colon cancer. Fiber occurs in whole grains, wheat and bran cereals, rice, popcorn, whole-wheat bread, fruits, and vegetables. Remember, some people do not tolerate a high-fiber diet well; they should be selective about which high-fiber foods to incorporate in their diet.

3. Choose foods with Vitamin A. Vitamin A is essential for healthy cell division. You can find plenty of Vitamin A in carrots, peaches, apricots, squash, and broccoli.

4. Do the same for Vitamin C. Vitamin C is essential for healthy cell metabolism and healthy cell walls. You'll find it naturally in fresh fruits and vegetables like grapefruit, cantaloupe, oranges, strawberries, red and green peppers, broccoli, and tomatoes.

5. Watch your weight. Keep your weight under control—eating neither too much nor too little. There is a tendency for the fat to get fatter and the thin to get thinner. Ideal weight plus a moderate exercise program maintains the cancer-fighting mechanisms of the body.

What Are the Risk Factors to Avoid?

1. Fat in your diet. A high-fat diet increases your risk of breast and colon cancer. Cut overall fat intake by eating lean meat, fish, skinned poultry, and low-fat dairy products. Avoid pastries and candies.

2. Salt-cured, smoked, nitrite-cured foods. Cancers of the esophagus and stomach are common in countries where these food are eaten in large quantities. Keep bacon, ham, hot dogs, or salt-cured fish to a minimum, or eliminate them entirely.

3. Tobacco—smoke or smokeless. Smoking is the biggest risk factor of all. This is the main cause of lung cancer and thirty percent of all cancers. Smokeless tobacco is the chief cause of cancer around the mouth and oro-pharynx.

4. Alcohol. If you drink a lot, your risk of cancer of the liver increases. Smoking and drinking alcohol increases your risk of cancer of the mouth, throat, voice box, and esophagus. Keep your alcohol intake to a minimum, or eliminate it entirely.

5. Sun. Too much sun causes skin cancer and other damage to your skin. Protect yourself with sunscreen and wear long sleeves and a hat during the midday hours, 11 A.M. to 3 P.M. Avoid indoor sunlamps and tanning parlors. If you notice changes in a mole or a sore that doesn't heal, *see your doctor immediately!*

MENTAL ATTITUDE

Bob Chapin of St. Petersburg, Florida, was told he had a fifty-fifty chance of surviving his cancer of the lymph system. Today, seven years later, Bob says, "I told my doctor I wasn't going to be in the fifty percent that doesn't make it." What made a difference in Bob's recovery? Part of it was his attitude: I will win over this disease.

The medical community is increasingly aware of the role a healthy mental attitude plays in recovery from all kinds of diseases, not just from cancer. Our minds and bodies function in complex interaction with each other. Anger, hostility, self-pity, and depression all tend to depress the immune system, something we'll look at more closely in the next part of this book. On the other hand a positive attitude like Bob's increases the possibility of a cure through medical treatments.

But a positive mental attitude is not in itself a cure. In a review of a book about cancer survivors, Dr. Norval F. Kemp rightly observes that "most physicians have developed a healthy respect for patients' mental attitude in relation to any disease." But Kemp also criticizes the book's antagonism to orthodox treatments and its view that "individual beliefs and attitudes are of *fundamental* importance in achieving a cure" (*Hospital & Health Services Administration,* v. 30, no. 5, p. 135, emphasis added).

If you browse in the medical section of a local bookstore, you'll find a surprising number of books that suggest you can cure your own cancer simply by adjusting your attitude. And they suggest a number of mental techniques.

For instance, one popular technique is called "visualizing." You find a quiet place, relax, and breathe deeply and regularly as your body relaxes. Then, when you are entirely relaxed, you mentally visualize the destruction and elimination of your cancer cells. Perhaps you suppose they are like minnows, and your white blood cells are predatory fish. You imagine the fish attacking and swallowing the frightened, swirling, and impotent cancer cells. Or if you're a hunter, you may imagine your immune system picking cancer cells off one by one, like clay pigeons. Any image that visualizes the good guys—your body's natural defenses—killing, destroying, eliminating the bad guys—your cancer—is supposed to enhance the capacity of the body to fight the disease. And this is because the mind is thought to control the body.

Now, it's true that studies have shown that athletes, by visualizing themselves performing their sports correctly, can "program" themselves physically to approximate the mental image. Experiments with college baseball players showed that a group assigned for two weeks to imagine themselves batting correctly improved their averages almost as much as those who took batting practice, while the averages of another group told to take the two weeks off declined. But battling cancer is no mind-over-matter phenomenon.

Just think about the difference between this and the many autonomic processes that take place in your body. You can lift your arm when you choose, but you don't have that kind of control over the flow of blood in your arm's vessels. You can blink your eyes, but its pupil size adjusts to light and darkness without your conscious control. You can lift your foot, but if you cut it, your blood will clot without you thinking about it. Literally millions of complex processes operate within your body every minute. Digestive juices flow, white blood cells attack disease-causing germs, the chemicals that cause your muscles to contract are used up and replaced—all this without any conscious effort on your part. In fact, most of these processes *can't* be directed by you, however you set your mind to it! Such processes may be *influenced* by such factors as your mental attitude. But they can't be controlled by you or anyone else.

It's this fact that troubles medical doctors about the growing enthusiasm for "self-induced healings" and for treating cancer by "attitude adjustment." There is some truth in the proponents' view of a link between positive attitude and good health. But a positive attitude is not the whole story. And, however positive your attitude may be, however actively you "visualize" your body's natural resources attacking your cancer, *you can't control your body's autonomic disease-fighting processes.*

Perhaps it would help if you thought of cancer treatment as something like a tuna casserole. There are a variety of ingredients in a casserole—tuna, mushroom soup, rice, lightly cooked green peas—all blended together in just the right proportions. It's the combination that makes the food both tasty and nutritious. If someone told you to leave out all the other ingredients and just eat the rice, you would know that wasn't right. The casserole needs all the ingredients.

While you're undergoing cancer treatments, you probably will run across at least one proponent of self-curing, some enthusiastic author who has survived cancer and believes that a positive mental attitude is everything. The person may even be a medical doctor. The cancer survivor will talk about the miraculous healing powers of the body and the mind, suggesting that if you adopt this or that mental technique, often supplemented by a "natural" diet, you can make yourself well without the help of surgery, chemotherapy, radiation, or the regular checkups offered by the medical community. And tragically, some people will believe it and abandon their life-saving medical treatments.

But when you read about or hear such a person, try to remember the tuna casserole. Yes, a positive mental attitude is a vital ingredient in conquering your cancer. But it's only *one* ingredient. Your mental attitude will indirectly affect your immune system and its ability to fight disease. But you can do nothing to control your body's battle with cancer.

I have tremendous respect for the powers of the human body to fight disease and illness. In my medical practice I've developed a deep appreciation for the intangibles. I've seen spontaneous remissions, medically unexplainable recoveries, and I've become sensitive to the tremendous contribution that a positive, determined attitude makes in fighting cancer. When you link that positive attitude to a balanced diet and follow the medically sound course of treatments prescribed by your doctor, you have the best chance of all to win over cancer. Chapter 7 will outline several other strategies to help you maintain a positive mental attitude.

SOMETHING TO DEPEND ON

When I treated Gloria, the Eurasian model who became so utterly depressed when I told her she needed a radical mastectomy, I worried about her negative attitude. I realized that her apathy and depression could seriously jeopardize her recovery from cancer. I told her that she needed to find something she could depend on, something that would give her support through this time.

As I bandaged her wound, I tried to give her some semblance of hope, any help in regaining a positive attitude. I explained what had worked for me, always adding, "Now, this may not make any sense to you." I told her about my relationship to the Lord, that no matter what time of the day or night I needed some help, I could draw on Christ as a source of help.

But I couldn't break through her silence. I felt as if I had failed, utterly. I had never run across someone as baffling as she was. Her intense withdrawal made me consider calling a psychiatrist to give me suggestions about how I could help her. A few weeks after surgery, her care was taken over by the oncologist, and I saw less of her. But her husband would call me once in a while and let me know what was going on. Her oncologist had started her on chemotherapy, and she had some troubles with that. But at least she had stayed in treatment. After chemotherapy Gloria went through a course of radiation.

Several years after her treatment, much to my surprise, Gloria called me and asked if she could see me. When she came for the appointment, I expected to see a really depressed woman.

Instead, into my office walked a radiant woman, dressed in a colorful dress and wide hat. Her whole person beamed.

The first thing she said to me was, "Meet your sister in Jesus." Gloria had found, as I had, that the Lord is a comfort and strength during our greatest trials. He had been her support in her fight with cancer. She went on, "You thought I didn't hear a word you said. But I heard every word. It got me through my surgery. It got me through my chemotherapy and my radiation. And I'm here for a reason. I want to start a support group for people who were in the same boat I was in."

That was some years ago. But as a result of her experience, Gloria launched Cancer Lifeline, a Seattle support network that remains very active in helping people get over their fear, anxieties, and uncertainties as they face their cancer.

This is one case where a woman who was really down found something to depend on—her faith in Jesus Christ— something that would help her get over the rough spots.

Dora is another patient who was treated for breast cancer.

When she learned she needed surgery, she was afraid she would lose her husband's love if her breast was removed. She could not face losing both a part of her body and her husband. Realizing the power of her fears, Dora's husband gave her constant encouragement. His response was, "Let's just get you well. When we do, we can have some fun. Go on trips and things."

Strengthened by her husband's support, Dora went into her surgery with a positive attitude. She was confident that her husband wanted *her*. The rest didn't matter. Dora went through her radical mastectomy very well. And she never fell back into her fear because her husband's love and acceptance continued to be a strong encouragement to her.

What I'm saying here is very simple. You need a foundation for your fight against cancer. You need a source of security, something or someone who won't let you down when things get rough.

You know, in recommending a personal relationship with God as the best foundation, I'm not suggesting that if you turn to him, your healing is guaranteed. The fact is that we're all terminal. We are all going to die—some sooner, some later. So religious faith isn't something you turn to in desperation, bargaining for a miracle. What many of my patients and I have found is that God provides the comfort of knowing we are loved even when life hurts and the confidence that in life or death, good things do lie ahead. It's that confidence that provides inner peace and serves as a firm foundation for the positive attitude that helps us fight, and often conquer, our disease.

QUESTIONS FOR THOUGHT
OR GROUP DISCUSSION

1. What does it mean to take control of your personal fight against cancer? What specific things can you do now to take more control?
2. What has characterized your own coping strategies in struggling with cancer up to this point?
3. What are some of the signs that indicate an unorthodox approach to treating cancer is potentially dangerous? Why is a person so vulnerable to the promises made by proponents of "natural" or "miracle" cancer cures? Have you felt tempted to take such a route yourself? If so, why? When were you most tempted?
4. What has given you or your family strength in your battle with cancer?
5. In the cancer diary in Part III of this book, I share a number of brief readings: poems, Scripture verses, and thoughts expressed by cancer patients. Find the ones most meaningful to you and use them as an aid to meditation when things are most difficult.

7

ON THE ROAD TO RECOVERY

The philosopher Plato recommended, "Know thyself." Much later a military man urged, "Know your enemy." Both are good advice for cancer patients.

The enemy, the disease, is a serious threat to life and health. To fight cancer effectively, you need to know certain things about the disease, about your particular cancer, and about how it may affect your lifestyle for the next few years. The more you know about your cancer and the more misunderstandings you can avoid, the better you'll be able to handle your situation.

Knowing yourself is important too. Fighting this disease will reveal inner resources you never realized you had. Sometimes you'll need help to develop those inner resources. But you *can* develop them. They'll not only help you in your fight against cancer, but they also will help you become a stronger person after your victory is won.

115

In this chapter I want to go over a few facts about cancer, to make sure you have information you'll need as you walk that sometimes long road to recovery. And I want to look at some sources of help you can draw on when things seem especially tough.

CANCER FACTS AND MYTHS

Cancer can strike anyone, at any time. Unfortunately, it kills more children aged three to fourteen than any other disease. And the older a person gets, the more prone he or she is to getting cancer. As our life expectancy increases, the incidence of cancer also increases. For example, American Cancer Society's *Cancer Facts and Figures 1990* reported that in the 1980s, 4.5 million people died from cancer and 9 million other people were diagnosed with cancer. Around 12 million people are currently under medical treatment for cancer. While that's a lot of people, here's what the future holds. About 78 million Americans now living will eventually have cancer. That's about 30 percent of our population. Over the years, cancer will strike approximately three out of four families.

You Can Survive

Yet there's a positive side. According to the same report, alive today in America are 6 million people who have had cancer, with 3 million of these considered cured (no evidence of the disease five years after its onset). What's more, the life expectancy of a person who has conquered cancer is the same as anyone who hasn't had the disease!

Of course, "cured" is a relative term. In my days of clinical medicine, I saw people whom I considered cured after one year, others after two or three years. It depends on the tumor, the patient, the treatment, and the physical signs. But one thing I do know. The figures are getting better all the time.

In 1900, few cancer patients had any hope of long-term survival. In the 1930s, less than one in five was alive after five years. In the 1940s, it was one in four, and in 1960, it was one in three. Today's figures are better, and even these are misleading. The American Cancer Society estimates that 42,500 of the cancer deaths that occurred in 1989 could have been avoided through early detection and treatment. And here's a shocking statistic: In 1989, 142,500 lives were lost from cancer—because of tobacco smoking.

The "Surviving Cancer" chart demonstrates that in almost every kind of cancer cited, the survival rate has gone up in the twelve-year period from 1974–1986—some as much as seven percent. And in the years since 1986, the rate has gone up even more.

The American Cancer Society reports that in 1990, total cancer deaths will be about 510,000—1,397 people a day. That's about one every minute. Yet subtract the almost 185,000 who will die unnecessarily because of late detection or continued smoking, and the figures are not as grim. Then subtract the unspecified number who will die because they gave up on proven medical treatments, and the facts support what I've been saying throughout this book. Today many cancer patients do have a realistic hope, not only of extending their lifetime but also of conquering cancer completely.

That hope is getting better all the time, as we'll see in Part II of this book. In the meantime, cancer is an enemy to respect, even though it is no longer the scourge that it was a decade or two ago.

You Can Take Precautions

Another edge cancer patients have today is the ability to combat cancer's recurrence. Recurrence worries people who

CONQUERING CANCER

SURVIVING CANCER AFTER 5 YEARS

Percentage of patients surviving five years after cancer was diagnosed, in five different groups of patients. For example, 66 percent of adults whose cancer was diagnosed from 1960 to 1963 were alive five years after the diagnosis.

Specific forms of cancer, all adults

	1974–76	1977–80	1981–86
CANCER SITES			
Oral cavity and pharynx	52.9%	52.0%	52.9%
Esophagus	4.7	5.2	8.0
Stomach	14.9	16.4	17.0
Colon	49.9	52.4	56.4
Rectum	48.1	49.6	53.4
Liver	3.8	2.9	4.5
Pancreas	2.7	2.6	3.1
Larynx	65.3	66.3	67.0
Lung and bronchus	12.2	13.1	13.1
Melanoma of skin	79.2	81.1	81.1
Breast	74.0	74.3	76.6
Cervix	68.3	67.3	65.8
Uterus	88.2	84.3	82.6
Ovary	36.5	38.0	38.9
Prostate gland	66.5	70.6	73.3
Testis	78.4	87.6	92.1
Urinary bladder	72.2	74.6	78.2
Kidney and renal pelvis	51.4	51.7	52.6
Brain and nervous system	22.1	24.2	24.8
Thyroid gland	91.8	92.5	94.2
Hodgkin's disease	70.9	73.1	75.9
Non-Hodgkin's lymphoma	46.9	48.2	50.8
Multiple myeloma	24.3	25.7	26.4
Leukemia	33.4	35.2	34.9

Adaptation of a chart published by the National Cancer Institute have or have had any cancer. Some cancers do recur—we'll look at that a little bit later. Let me assure you though, the longer you remain free of your cancer after your initial treatment, the more that fear will fade. What should not fade is your awareness of the precautions you need to take to avoid other cancers or to detect them early enough so they can be successfully treated.

1. *See your doctor if you observe any of cancer's early warning signs and have regular checkups.* The "Cancer Checkup Chart" lists those early signs and identifies periodic exams the American Cancer Society recommends people should have for cancer detection. During your recovery period you'll have more frequent checkups. But after you've been considered "cured," you'll want to follow this or a more frequent schedule of checkups.

2. *Rigorously eliminate known cancer risks from your lifestyle.* Today no one doubts the relationship between smoking and lung cancer. A short twenty years ago, many doubted that cause-effect link. I can remember attending medical conventions where the air was blue with smoke. Today it would be unthinkable to light up a cigarette in such a meeting. The act would be totally—and actively!—rejected. Our society is making progress. Restaurants have no-smoking sections. Many airline flights are smoke free. We've begun to realize that smokeless areas are important in the workplace, because even secondhand smoke is carcinogenic (can cause cancer). The more rigorously you eliminate tobacco smoke from your life, the better your chance will be of living free of lung cancer. By the way, some people in our society claim that marijuana smoke is "clean" and not responsible for lung

CONQUERING CANCER

CANCER CHECKUP CHART

See your doctor if you observe any of these cancer danger signals:

1. Unusual bleeding or discharge
2. A lump that doesn't go away
3. A sore that doesn't heal within two weeks
4. A change in bowel or bladder habits
5. Persistent hoarseness or cough
6. Indigestion or difficulty in swallowing
7. Change in a wart or mole

See your doctor for regular, periodic exams to detect early cancers.

Test	Patient Age	Frequency*
Breast self-exam	over 20	Monthly
Breast physical exam	20–40 over 40	Every 3 years Annually
Digital rectal exam	over 40	Annually
Endometric tissue exam	at menopause	
Mammography	35–40 40–49 over 50	One baseline Every 1, 2 years Annually
Pap smear	20–65	2 consecutive years normal report, then every 3 years
Sigmoidoscopy	Over 50	2 consecutive years normal exam, then every 3–5 years
Stool guaiac	Over 50	Annually

*During recovery from a cancer, scheduled exams will be much more frequent and will often include additional tests. Your doctor will develop a follow-up schedule, which you will want to follow carefully.

cancer. The evidence just isn't on their side. The incidence of cancer from pot smoke is the same as from tobacco smoke.

A second risk comes from the sun. Not long ago, a dark suntan was a mark of beauty and appeal. People would bake out in the sun, trying their best to outdo friends. However, our values have changed. Now that we know that excessive sun exposure injures skin layers and predisposes us to some forms of cancer, we take precautions—sunblockers, hats, shading devices—against destructive sun exposure.

A third cancer risk is radiation. The first time I encountered skin cancer was in my internship, when I saw the hands of a radiologist who had carelessly done years of hand-held fluoroscopy (a diagnostic tool that uses direct exposure by X rays) and had subjected his hands to X rays. Unfortunately, the effect of X-ray exposure is cumulative. The amount of radiation my friend had received was at a severely damaging level. His hands were dry from the destruction of normal oil glands and crusted with emerging cancer spots. Before long he was forced to quit practice, and his hands lost their ability to function.

Today there's no excuse for exposing yourself to tobacco, excessive sun rays, or radiation. By eliminating these from your lifestyle, you can go a long way toward preventing the recurrence of an old cancer or the development of a new one.

3. Maintain good general health. The AIDS epidemic has heightened public awareness of the importance of our immune system. The AIDS virus attacks the immune system, weakening it and making the body easy prey to other diseases. Most AIDS patients die not from the AIDS virus itself but from the body's inability to fight off other infections.

A deficient immune system also can lead to certain cancers, such as Kaposi's sarcoma. To give yourself every chance of fighting off the disease, you need to maintain general good health. This means watching your diet, your exercise, and your sleep.

An article in a popular magazine recently claimed that about one third of all cancer deaths may be related to the food we eat. The only way that statement would not be misleading is if "may be" were underlined, italicized, and followed by about a dozen question marks. Despite the popular notion that certain foods can be blamed for causing cancer or for keeping the body from fighting cancer, no scientific proof for such a claim exists.

But a healthy diet, with plenty of fiber and reduced fat, can help us ward off cancer. The National Cancer Institute recommends eating more grains to increase fiber and more low-fat meat, poultry, and fish. It also recommends roasting or baking foods rather than frying them. And it's always important to eat a balanced diet, like the diet described in chapter 6.

As for exercise, you don't have to run the marathon to maintain good muscle tone and strengthen your cardiovascular system. A good brisk walk each day will do. During your recovery period, that walk may be quite short. But making the effort to go a little way, and then a little farther, will pay off.

BE REALISTIC AND HOPEFUL

One of the greatest fears of any cancer patient is that the cancer will spread or recur. Even if you take recommended treatments, eat properly, and maintain a positive attitude, this can happen. But even the spread of a cancer, or its recurrence after treatment, isn't necessarily a sentence of doom. I know it's discouraging. But for some of us the fight against cancer is long and hard.

ON THE ROAD TO RECOVERY

I can't tell you whether your cancer battle will be quick and easy or long and hard. But I can cite statistics to give you an idea of what you may be up against. If you have a serious cancer, you need to know up front that you've got a real battle on your hands. So I've provided a brief summary classification of cancers, by bodily system (skin cancers, cancers of the digestive system, etc.). Locate the "Classification of Cancers by System" chart, and when you've found your cancer, run your finger across the chart. Here's the data you'll find and how to use it.

System and organ. This merely identifies and locates the tumor.

Cell type. This helps classify the tumor as to the general makeup of the cancer. For example, cancer of the bowel usually arises in the lining of the bowel, which makes it carcinoma. If it were to arise from another layer of the bowel, however, it could be either a sarcoma or a lymphoma.

Risk factors. This identifies factors that make it more likely a person will develop this kind of cancer. Although it's almost impossible to determine the causes of cancers, it is possible to determine what factors place a person at risk for a particular cancer. (For example, excessive exposure to the sun makes it more likely that a person will develop one of the skin cancers.) You can use the information in this column to reduce your risk of recurrence. For instance, stay out of the sun during the hottest part of the day and use a sunscreen to reduce risk of skin cancer.

Seriousness. The asterisks (*) in this column indicate how formidable the cancer is in terms of difficulty of treatment and likelihood of recurrence. A single asterisk (*) indicates a limited threat. At the other end of the scale, five asterisks (*****) indicate a very serious threat. Please remember that even if your cancer has a five-asterisk rating, this doesn't mean you have no hope. It simply means that you need to prepare yourself for a long struggle.

Symptoms. Symptoms are what you experience: they are what you feel, notice, and report to your doctor. For instance, symptoms of skin cancer may include a flaking or crusty spot that slowly becomes larger. Symptoms of another cancer may be nagging pain that doesn't go away or persistent weight loss. It's important to report any of the symptoms mentioned in this column to your doctor when you notice them.

Signs and diagnostic tests. Signs are the physical cancer indicators that your doctor observes when he or she examines you. In an easily accessible area like the skin, cancer signs and signals are both visible to the eye. In other areas, you may report your symptoms (how you feel), but your doctor will need to conduct tests to discover hidden signs. The information in this column tells you the signs the doctor will look for in order to confirm or rule out a diagnosis of cancer. The common diagnostic tests are cited. These include such things as biopsy, X ray, blood tests, scopes, CT, MRI, and ultrasound.

Likelihood of spread. This column indicates how slowly or how rapidly a cancer spreads. Growth is rated from a single asterisk (*) indicating very slow growth, to five asterisks (*****) for extremely fast-spreading cancers. Some cancers tend to spread more than others. In addition, while some cancers only spread locally, other cancers spread to adjacent organs or even distant parts of the body. For example, a basal cell skin cancer rarely spreads to other parts of the body, while a melanoma often does.

Treatment. This column identifies the treatment(s) you can expect to receive for your cancer. To find out more about any of the three major treatment types, reread chapters 3, 4, or 5.

Prognosis. This predicts the outcome of the tumor in a general way. I hesitate to include this category, simply because it's so easily misunderstood. This is a *statistical* category. It lumps everyone with a particular kind of cancer in one big group and looks at how many of them are likely to die from that kind of cancer. I'm always troubled by such statistics because they fail to consider several factors. They don't consider your general health, your attitude, your lifestyle, or the many other personal factors that affect recovery. Even if a particular cancer typically claims 90 percent of the people who develop it, this doesn't mean that *you* will be one of the 90 percent. You may just as well be one of the 10 percent who survive!

In this column, a five-asterisk rating (*****) is good news, for it means that 95–100 percent of such cancers will be eradicated. On the other hand a one-asterisk rating (*) means that you must prepare to fight for your life. That rating does *not* mean that you should give up. There is always, always, reason to hope.

Now one more word about recurrence. As you complete your treatments, your doctor will establish a follow-up schedule. Typically you'll go back to your family doctor for follow-up, rather than continue with your oncologist, surgeon, or radiologist. A follow-up program has three important goals: First, to detect any recurrence of the primary

CLASSIFICATION OF CANCERS BY SYSTEM

System and Organ	Cell Type	Risk Factors	Seriousness	Symptoms	Signs and Diagnostic Tests	Likelihood of Spread	Treatment	Prognosis
SKIN	basal cell	chronic sun exposure	*	small scaly area that does not heal, bleeds easily	crusted, ulcerated, pearly borders	*	excision biopsy	*****
	squamous cell	chronic sun exposure or old sunburn scar	**	small scaly area that does not heal, bleeds easily	crusted, ulcerated, no pearly borders	**	excision biopsy	****, if treated early
	malignant melanoma	chronic sun exposure	*****	changing black mole	black mole, irregular borders, satellite tiny black spots. excision biopsy	*****	staging, grading, wide excision. watch for regional nodes	**
DIGESTIVE SYSTEM lip	carcinoma	chronic sun exposure, pipe smoking	**	non-healing, sore lower lip	hardened ulcer, biopsy	***	excision	****
mouth	carcinoma	chronic irritation, smokeless tobacco	***	enlarging ulcer	ulcer, biopsy	***	excision	***

tongue	carcinoma	chronic irritation, tobacco	****	painful, non-healing sore	hardened ulcer with ragged borders, biopsy	***	excision, radiation if extended	***, if treated early
salivary gland (parotid)	carcinoma	unknown	**	slow-growing lump in front of ear	mass in tail of parotid gland	**	biopsy, surgical radiation	***
pharyngeal (back of throat)	carcinoma	unknown	*****	sore throat, painful swallowing, streaks of blood	ulcer behind tongue, biopsy	****	surgery, radiation	*
esophageal	carcinoma	unknown	*****	none, to some difficulty swallowing	ulcerating mass seen by esophagoscope, X ray, biopsy	****	surgery, radiation, chemotherapy	*
stomach	carcinoma, sarcoma	unknown	*****	pain, indigestion, weight loss	ulcerating mass seen by X ray, gastroscope	****	surgery, radiation, chemotherapy	*
pancreatic	carcinoma	unknown	*****	weight loss, jaundice, pain	GI scan, ultrasound, laparoscopy	*****	extensive surgery, chemotherapy	*
gall bladder	carcinoma	unknown	*****	pain, jaundice	X ray, ultrasound, laparoscopy	*****	surgery, chemotherapy, radiation	*

System and Organ	Cell Type	Risk Factors	Seriousness	Symptoms	Signs and Diagnostic Tests	Likelihood of Spread	Treatment	Prognosis
DIGESTIVE SYSTEM								
liver	carcinoma	alcohol, benzine (solvent)	*****	nausea, vomiting, weight loss, loss of appetite	enlarged liver diagnosed by X ray, CT scan, ultrasound, needle biopsy	****	surgery, chemotherapy	**
small intestine	carcinoma	unknown	****	weight loss, cramps, blood in stool, diarrhea	difficult to diagnose, X ray sometimes used	****	surgery, radiation, chemotherapy	*
large intestine—cecum (right colon)	carcinoma	unknown	**	blood in stool, anemia	blood in stool, right abdominal mass seen by X ray, colonoscope, ultrasound	**	surgery	***
large intestine—recto-sigmoid (left colon)	carcinoma	unknown	***	blood in stool, constipation	sigmoidoscope, barium enema, colonoscope	**	surgery, radiation if necessary	****

RESPIRATORY SYSTEM								
nasal turbinates	carcinoma	cocaine, snuff	****	bloody discharge, obstruction	inflammation, ulceration	***	radiation	*
sinuses (ethmoid, frontal, maxillary)	carcinoma	unknown	****	pain, drainage	dull illumination, X-ray shadows	**	surgery and X ray	*
naso-pharyngeal	carcinoma	smoking	*****	bloody sputum	ulcer, biopsy	***	radiation	*
laryngeal (voice box)	carcinoma	smoking	*****	hoarseness, cough, blood	vocal-cord lesion, biopsy	***	surgery, radiation	**
bronchogenic (lung)—starts in bronchial tubes and most often spreads to lungs	carcinoma	smoking	****	persistent cough, bloody sputum, weight loss	cancer cells recovered by bronchoscopy, X ray, CT	****	surgery, radiation, chemotherapy	*
CARDIO-VASCULAR	Cancers of the heart or blood vessels are very rare.							
GENITO-URINARY								
kidney	renal cell	unknown	****	bloody urine, pain	flank mass, bloody urine, X ray, CT	***	surgery, radiation, chemotherapy	**

System and Organ	Cell Type	Risk Factors	Seriousness	Symptoms	Signs and Diagnostic Tests	Likelihood of Spread	Treatment	Prognosis
GENITO-URINARY								
bladder	transitional cell, squamous cell	unknown aniline dyes, chemicals, tobacco	**	frequent urination, bloody urine	mass seen by cytoscope, biopsy	**	surgery, frequent re-examination	***
penile (penis)	carcinoma	rare, but very serious when it occurs	****	ulcerated sore	biopsy	***	surgery	***
testicular (testis)	seminoma, chorio carcinoma	unknown	**	pain, tenderness, enlargement	inflammation, tender mass	****	surgery, radiation	****
prostatic (prostate)	carcinoma	unknown	**	increasing difficulty in urination	biopsy, firm mass on rectal examination	**	surgery, hormones	***
ovarian	serous cystadeno carcinoma, Brenner's Tumor	unknown	****	mass, pain	pelvic mass, ultrasound	***	surgery, chemotherapy	**
uterine	carcinoma	unknown	***	irregular bleeding	D & C	**	surgery, radiation	**

cervical	carcinoma	irritation, infection, human papilloma virus	**	bleeds easily	cervicitis, tested by Pap smear, biopsy	**	surgery, radiation	****
vulval (vulva)	carcinoma	rare, serious when it occurs	*****	non-healing skin lesion	biopsy	****	surgery, radiation	**
NEURO-LOGICAL brain	Brain cells do not divide, so any cancer of the "brain" is a cancer of the supportive tissues of the brain.							
	hemangioma, glioma, astrocytoma, meningioma	unknown	****	dizziness, paralysis, seizures	X ray, MRI	**	surgery	*
	acoustic neuroma	unknown	**	vertigo, hearing loss	X ray, MRI	**	surgery	****
BONE MARROW	acute myelogenous leukemia	unknown	*****	anemia, fever, fatigue	abnormal white blood count, bone marrow	***	chemotherapy, marrow transplant	*
	chronic lymphocytic leukemia	unknown	**	anemia, weakness	white blood count, bone marrow	**	chemotherapy	***
	multiple myeloma	unknown	****	anemia, weakness	bone marrow analysis	**	chemotherapy	*

System and Organ	Cell Type	Risk Factors	Seriousness	Symptoms	Signs and Diagnostic Tests	Likelihood of Spread	Treatment	Prognosis
IMMUNE SYSTEM	Hodgkin's disease	unknown	**	none, to fever, enlarged nodes, fatigue	enlarged nodes, biopsy	***	radiation, chemotherapy	***
	lymphoma, lymphosarcoma	unknown	***	none, to mass, weakness, fever	biopsy, careful staging and grading	**	surgery, chemotherapy, radiation	***
ENDOCRINE SYSTEM thyroid	carcinoma	exposure to radiation	**	mass	mass, abnormal lab or X-ray findings	**	surgery, medication, I_{131} radiation	***
adrenal cortex	carcinoma	unknown	****	virilization in women, feminization in men	abnormal development, abnormal male and female sex hormones, CT	***	surgery, radiation	**

MUSCULO-SKELETAL SYSTEM								
bone	osteogenic sarcoma	unknown	****	pain, inflammation	X ray	***	surgery, chemotherapy	**
muscle and ligament	rhabdomyosar-coma	unknown	***	painful mass, extremity	tender mass, X ray, biopsy	***	surgery, chemotherapy	**
EYE	melanoma	unknown	****	decreased vision	diagnosed by examination	*****	high energy X ray, enucleation	***

tumor so that it can be treated in its earliest and least-threatening stage; second, to detect any other malignancies that develop; third, to provide emotional support and help you face any new threat.

Every cancer holds some risk of recurrence. In most sites, if the cancer does recur, it will do so within five years of the original therapy. In the case of breast cancer, most recurrences take place within the first two years after treatment, although some risk exists for twenty or thirty years. On the other hand, in the case of colon or rectal cancer that does not penetrate the muscularis (muscular wall), the risk of recurrence in five years is less than five percent. The doctor's follow-up schedule will take these things into account and be structured for your specific case.

Cancer recurrence expresses itself in several ways. A *local* recurrence means the cancer has come back at or near its original site. A *regional* recurrence means a new tumor has grown in lymph nodes or tissues near the original site. And a *metastatic* recurrence means the original cancer has spread to distant organs or tissues. Doctors can often recognize a metastatic cancer by examining the cancer-cell structure for similarities with the cells found in the original site. The important thing is to make sure you have regular follow-up examinations and remember that recurrences, like original cancers, can be treated.

A recurrence is a setback, obviously. But most often that's all it is. You still have plenty of reasons to hope.

FACING CANCER'S DOWNSIDE

"I feel sorry," Jacqueline Fenton said, "because I don't want to die young and leave my family. But these are things that are going to happen. If I have to deal with something like that, I want to do it in a positive way. First of all, I don't want to spoil the time I have by being angry. And second of all, I have always been a fairly happy and content person, and I am not going to go out of this world leaving them with a different image."

Jackie Fenton's story was told in Canada's *Maclean's* magazine of June 13, 1988. In October of 1984, the doctors removed a two-inch malignant tumor from her left breast and two days later they removed the entire breast. Then in April of 1986, Jackie developed a persistent rib pain that the doctors diagnosed as cancer of one rib. Her cancer had returned and spread. In May, specialists began radiation treatments. By March 1987, her cancer had spread to her lungs. A year later, in March 1988, a bone scan revealed that the cancer had spread throughout her body. She resumed chemotherapy, this time primarily to ease her pain. And she said at that time, "I'm not talking any more about living for years. It's more down to months."

This is cancer's major downside. Cancer is a killer, and despite the fact that many of its victims recover, far too many will surely die of their disease.

I have been optimistic and upbeat throughout this book and honestly so. Many cancers can be successfully treated today. And I encourage you to hope. But some people with cancer are going to lose their battle. If, despite everything you and your doctors can do, you should be one of those people, you're going to discover you have unexpected inner resources. Just as Jacqueline Fenton did.

First, she found the inner strength to *face reality*. Pretending won't drive the prospect of death away, and it will keep us from finding inner peace.

Second, she found the inner strength to *enjoy each remaining day* of her life. She and her husband took vacations during breaks in her treatments. They visited friends and spent time with her two young grandchildren.

Third, she found the inner strength to *maintain and strengthen relationships,* especially her relationship to her husband. Often as the years and months of struggling with cancer near an end, a person finds renewed intimacy in his or her most important relationships.

Fourth, she found the inner strength to *achieve a tranquil acceptance.* "Sometimes when I'm in church and it's very solemn," she said, "I will think of my children, and the tears will come, and they are very hard to stop. But there is nothing brave about what I'm doing. When you have to do it, you don't have any choice. I've been given a very good life, and I have enjoyed it."

For me, another reality makes death, though an enemy, less than fearsome. I simply can't believe that when the body dies, all that you are—that essential "you" that is absolutely unique—simply ends. I truly believe that human beings are made in the image of God and are precious to him. For me, the proof of that is found in Jesus, who died for our sins and then was raised from the dead. Christ's resurrection is my guarantee. I know that when death strips me of this life, there's a new and better life awaiting me with the Lord.

This faith sustained me during my own fight with cancer. I've seen it sustain hundreds of my patients throughout the years. And I've seen this faith, that's anchored in the Bible rather than in wishful thinking, help many terminally ill patients find peace.

A TOUGH FIGHT AHEAD

Another real concern is the lengthy struggle many cancers cause. No fight with cancer is easy. Sometimes a therapy will make you feel so sick you wish you *could* die! And certainly cancer will cause many adjustments. But it's during this struggle that you'll discover inner resources that will strengthen you. Despite discouragement and setbacks, you'll get up and face the next day with quiet courage. You'll keep on. And I pray that you'll win.

Several things will help you develop your inner resources.

1. Seek loving support from your family. One of the good things about cancer is that it's not contagious. In other words, it's impossible to transfer the malignant cells from one person to another. So there's no need to worry about intimacy with your loved ones. You can hug and be hugged. You can kiss and be kissed. You can continue an intimate relationship with your spouse. You can be absolutely certain that no one will "catch" the disease from you.

2. Take advantage of counseling help. Many cancer patients need two kinds of counseling help: practical counseling and supportive counseling. Practical counseling helps patients deal with issues like the financial impact of cancer or the possible loss of time at work. Supportive counseling helps them deal with the emotional impact of the disease. In my experience, the best source for each of these kinds of counseling is the hospital where you receive your treatment. Most cancer units have social workers who are familiar with community resources and who provide the practical guidance. And most cancer units also sponsor small support groups or offer individual supportive counseling help. Or you may be directed to one of the many cancer support groups sponsored by national or local organizations.

CANCER SUPPORT GROUPS

The Cancer Information Service	1-800-4-CANCER
I CAN COPE	1-212-736-3030
MAKE TODAY COUNT, INC.	1-314-348-1619
CANSURMOUNT	1-212-736-3030

When you look for a counselor or support group, be sure to choose carefully. You may want to work through your oncologist to find reputable organizations. Or rely on the personal recommendation of someone you know. The important thing is to find a place where you feel comfortable and receive the help you need.

And don't overlook the warm support provided by pastors and congregations of many local churches. It's particularly comforting to know that you have the prayer support of believing friends.

3. Try to live as normal a life as possible. Even if you're in the hospital, surround yourself with familiar things. A comfortable pair of shoes, a favorite casual outfit, a picture or vase on the bedstand. When you're home, you'll find your strength limited, so set daily priorities. Do the things you find most enjoyable or satisfying. If you're able to work at your job full time, fine. If not, and your work is important to you, perhaps you can work part time. Accept the limitations placed on you by your treatments or the particular stage of the disease, but remain active within those limits.

4. Set realistic, short-term goals. It really helps if you have some way to measure progress in your fight with cancer. The progress doesn't have to be great to be meaningful and satisfying. When you're really sick, a goal such as, "I'm going to sit up for a whole hour," or "I'm going to walk out and look at my flowerbed" is enough. As your recovery continues, set more difficult goals to achieve.

Many people find it helpful to keep a diary or journal during their treatment and recovery time. You may want to start one too. Record in it your progress, symptoms, goals, hopes, dreams, and fears. Jot down the kind things people say to you and do for you during this time. Occasionally read over your entries, noting your progress.

I kept a diary during my cancer experience. I recorded in it not only my feelings and reflections but also Scripture verses, personal stories, and medical articles. I found strength in meditating on the verses and poems, and I found a release in writing down my thoughts and feelings. I certainly didn't write in it every day—some days I didn't feel well enough even to think about it—but I did what I could. I've included that diary in Part III of this book. I've reworked it some and organized the entries into the emotional stages cancer patients often move through: disbelief, isolation, uncertainty, resignation, courage, searching, comfort, growing confidence, stretching, setting goals, sensitivity, and thankfulness.

Your diary may not be anything like mine, but I can promise that it will be valuable to you. Later on, you will appreciate reading some of the insights you gained while you were facing tough times. You will be amazed to see your progress. And you will be overwhelmed to read about the loving things people did for you.

5. Cultivate thankfulness and appreciation. I found in battling my cancer that I became especially sensitive to nature. I watched birds with a new appreciation. Even the wind in the trees, the warmth of the afternoon sun, and the color of the sky awakened a sense of thankfulness. I realized that I was surrounded by beauty and was even glad that I had been forced to take time out from my busy life to enjoy it.

It's all too easy when struggling with a disease like cancer to focus too much on ourselves and our feelings. Looking outside ourselves, sensing and being thankful for the beauty around us, is an important source of inner strength.

6. *Draw on religious faith.* When our lives are threatened, we have to go back to basics. If you have a religious faith, now is the time to draw on it. If not, now is a good time to consider some of life's basic questions. I've seen a lot of people who lived for material possessions and were tremendously successful. But when their lives were threatened, they realized all those things they had collected weren't much help.

Alcoholics Anonymous has demonstrated that when a person runs into a problem he or she can't handle, that person needs the help of a higher power. I've seen the same thing in my forty years as a physician and have experienced it in my own life. Turning things over to God, trusting yourself and your future to him, is a truly important source of inner strength in your battle with cancer.

"CURED"

I've written about death as cancer's downside. That's the worst but not the only long-term impact cancer can have on your life.

Jerry, a doctor who was an active skier and tennis player, developed a tumor in his leg. The tumor turned out to be a rhabdomyosarcoma, which is a highly malignant tumor. In the early days of cancer treatment—say in the forties or fifties—this kind of tumor would certainly have meant amputation for Jerry. However, with today's technology, the doctors decided to do extensive surgery to remove the tumor and the surrounding muscle and nerve. The surgery was so extensive that during the post-operative course, Jerry was totally out of work and totally disabled.

Before he went to surgery, he was not outwardly fearful, just stunned. He was quite anxious about his future work as a doctor. He was also afraid his sports activity was finished—which it was. At his wife's request, I went to see Jerry at his home. It was obvious that he was doing very well despite intensive chemotherapy. Jerry's wife was his support during this time, and she was terrific. He gradually has regained his ambulation, to the point that he no longer uses a cane. And his attitude has changed so he doesn't even give his disability a thought now, some three or four years later. He's totally recovered, and his prognosis is very positive.

Other than a period when Jerry was depressed and uncertain about his future, he adapted remarkably well. I saw him just the other day, and except for a slight limp, he seemed back to normal, kidding and joking as he usually did.

Jerry's experience reminds us that the battle with cancer can be a long one. Even when we win over the disease, it can cause some long-term changes in our lifestyle. But Jerry's experience also tells me that, despite the temporary dips and the changes cancer may make in our lives, as the years pass, we can look back and realize that we are our old selves again. Perhaps you may have a permanent reminder—something like Jerry's limp—that stays with you. But life will go on, and as it does, deep down you'll be a stronger and better person than you were.

Now that we've discussed the diagnosis and various treatments of cancer, we'll explore in Part II three other significant areas that will give you even more hope: understanding cancer cells, understanding how your immune system works, and becoming aware of the incredible advances in both cancer research and cancer treatment—advances that will help you conquer your cancer.

QUESTIONS FOR THOUGHT
OR GROUP DISCUSSION

1. What are the inner resources you've discovered you have during your or your loved one's battle with cancer?
2. What cancer facts in this chapter help you remain hopeful that your cancer will be cured?
3. What can you learn about your cancer itself? See the "Classification of Cancer by System" chart for basic information. See the selected bibliography at the end of this book. And ask your doctor for suggestions and more specific information.
4. If cancer gets a terminal grip, which of the suggestions for facing cancer's "downside" seems most helpful?
5. Take the first step in becoming involved in a cancer support group (if you're not already involved). Phone a local support network. If you're not aware of any group, ask your oncologist or people at your hospital to recommend an effective support group that will help you with emotional support and practical guidance for dealing with financial and other difficulties associated with cancer. Then follow through and make contact.

PART II

The Promise of Tomorrow

8

UNDERSTANDING CANCER CELLS

In 1987, a technique with great promise for conquering cancer was used in Leicester, England, to solve two rape murders. Blood and semen taken from two teenage victims indicated that the person who killed the first girl was the same person who killed the second one. Dr. Alec Jeffreys, a geneticist (a person who studies the parts of our cells that pass on hereditary traits) who learned to "read" parts of the distinct pattern stamped on each person's individual cells, had developed a process now called "genetic fingerprinting." Jeffreys used the blood samples to identify specific characteristics of the killer's genetic pattern, a pattern indelibly stamped on every cell in the killer's body. The killer's genetic characteristics were then compared with those of 4,000 men who fit a police profile of the likely killer. When one man got a co-worker to give blood in his name, he was arrested, tested—and found to have the matching genetic fingerprint. Faced with this evidence, the man confessed.

What does the forensic use of genetic fingerprinting have to do with conquering cancer? Genetic fingerprinting is possible only because each cell in a person's body contains his or her unique code, stamped in the center of every cell and recorded in genes and chromosomes. (If you don't understand what genes and chromosomes are, stay with me. The next several pages should help you understand some basic things about them.) Each individual's code, which exists from conception, is like a blueprint of the mature adult. This genetic code spells out things like color and thickness of hair, body shape and size, disposition to gain weight, the shape of ears, noses, and eyebrows—every distinct quality that makes one human body different from all others.

But something else is also set by the code: personal weaknesses. And one of these weaknesses is a propensity to develop cancer. *The key to understanding cancer's cause (and cure) lies in the genetic material found in every cell of your body.*

Today hundreds of scientists are focusing on a study of what is called the human *genome,* a term formed from the two words "*gene*" and "chromos*ome.*" Articles featuring new discoveries are already appearing in popular magazines and newspapers, and medical reporters feature them on radio and television reports. Many of these articles promise the total conquest of cancer.

My goal in this part of the book is to give you background information that will help you understand articles and reports about cancer research and its implications for conquering cancer. The concepts we'll look at aren't easy to grasp. The study of the human genome is unbelievably complex. But you can understand the basics and master enough of the terminol-

ogy to help you trace the emergence of a cancer-free future as
it unfolds.

THE SOURCE OF EACH PERSON'S
GENETIC CODE

To put everything in perspective, we need to go back to the
beginning of each person's life, when a male sperm and a
female ovum unite to form a single-celled organism called a
zygote. Although the zygote is a large cell, it is barely visible to
the naked eye. This single cell multiplies again and again. As it
does, tissues differentiate: that is, nerves, bones, muscles, and
organs form. And the code that controls all this development
lies at the center of every single cell. As the cell divides, it
passes on the genetic code to each new cell.

In one sense the human genetic code is shared by all of us:
the human being is designed to have two arms, two legs, one
head, ten fingers, one heart, and so on. In another sense, the
code that carries all your traits is individualized, different in
significant ways for each person. All humans have a face, but
people differ in size and length of nose, the shape of the
mouth, the color of the eyes, and so on.

Our special, personal genetic code is created through a truly
fascinating process. To trace that process, we might begin
with the sperm, the male sex cell. Many billions of immature
sperm cells lie dormant in the testicle, waiting their turn to
mature and be released into the apex of the female vagina
during sexual intercourse.

It takes seventy-four days for an infant sperm to mature to
the point at which it can fertilize an ovum. The process that
prepares the sperm for reproduction is called *meiosis*, which is
the first step in setting the genetic code.

The first change in a round, immature sperm is division of

the single, forty-six-chromosome cell into two cells, each with twenty-three chromosomes. Then a second change takes place. The chromosomes split down the middle, mix and shuffle themselves, and in the process end up with four mature sperm, each with twenty-three chromosomes. Two of these sperm have the X chromosome (which carry female characteristics), and two have the Y chromosome (which carry male characteristics).

Once the sperm is deposited at the apex of the vagina, it makes its way toward the ovum. The first sperm to reach the ovum fires an enzyme, and the ovum's cell membrane opens and allows that sperm in. The membrane closes immediately and will not let any other sperm in even though they fire the same enzyme.

The ovum, 1000 times as large as the sperm, consists of a cell membrane, a nucleus containing chromosomes, and cytoplasm, which provides nourishment. Once the sperm enters the ovum, the ovum's twenty-three chromosomes unite with the sperm's twenty-three chromosomes—and a unique new cell is created. That cell carries all the genetic traits of the mother and father, as well as those of generations of grandparents. Yet the genetic material has combined in a way that, from the very beginning, launches the life of a totally unique human being.

The blueprint of every trait of the mature person, from hair color to bone structure, from intelligence to temperament is laid down in that initial combination of genes and chromosomes at conception. In a very real sense, the mature adult is present in the fertilized egg.

And there too lies the key to cancer's cause—and cure. A truth we've discovered and only begun to understand.

UNDERSTANDING CANCER CELLS

GENES, CHROMOSOMES, AND DNA

Until recently no one had a way to study the inner structure of any cell. It was only in 1953 that Dr. James Watson and Dr. Francis Crick discovered that the substance at the center of the cell is *deoxyribonucleic acid* (DNA). In 1962, in the center of the Seattle World's Fair science building, I saw a mock-up model of the DNA molecule found in a particular virus. I had read about DNA, and as I stood before the huge model, I was amazed at the complexity and impressiveness of the chemical nature of that relatively simple DNA molecule.

Today with the aid of photoelectron microscopes, X-ray diffraction, and other tools, we are able to study the very building blocks of life. We know that all living cells, including bacteria and viruses, are dependent on DNA for their existence, function, and ability to replicate. Without DNA there is no life.

A lot more has been learned about DNA. The DNA molecule has been described as two ladders, placed side by side, but in opposite directions, and then twisted like a corkscrew, and finally wrapped tightly together to form a ball. Within this framework are billions of atoms, which look like very tight clusters of grapes. If we unwound that ball, we would find that the DNA molecule could be up to nine feet long, yet it is only 1/1000 of the thickness of the tiniest spiderweb filament. If all the DNA in the human body was laid end to end, it would reach to the moon and back nearly 8,000 times! And it's here, within the DNA, that the chromosomes and genes of the living creature are found.

The forty-six chromosomes in each human cell carry 100,000 genes, each made of protein chains formed by combinations of twenty different amino acids containing four

149

different subunits, called *nucleotides,* of which there are more than three billion in each cell. That's complex!

People have struggled to find analogies to express how complicated the human genome really is. Here's the best I've found. Suppose that each molecule in a strand of DNA is represented by a single letter. Suppose, then, that we print the letters, in the sequence the molecules appear, to represent the code of one person's DNA. That code would fill the thirty-two-volume *Encyclopedia Britannica* approximately thirteen times! Stop and think about that.

In the past decade microbiologists using new tools and techniques have been able to describe the complexity of the human DNA molecule. In fact, a seventy-four-foot model of a DNA chain is located at the Epcot Center's "Future World" pavilion featuring human life and health.

THE DIFFERENCE YOUR DNA MAKES

I've explained how the genes and chromosomes you inherited from your two parents, mixed together in a fresh, new pattern, make you a unique person. The genes control your hair color, your eye color, determine your potential height and intelligence, and so on. We now know that many hidden, organic traits are also genetically determined. We know certain diseases are inherited and have little to do with any choices we may make ourselves.

One example is cholesterol metabolism. If you haven't inherited an adequate amount of a certain gene, called the *apogene,* it will be almost impossible for you to have a normal cholesterol level. You'll have a much higher risk of heart disease than the person who has inherited enough of that preventive gene. That's the reason one person can eat a fairly high-cholesterol diet and have a normal level, while another person on a very low-cholesterol diet comes up with a high cholesterol count.

That doesn't seem quite fair. And it isn't. But that's the way it is. Each of us inherits a different deck of cards, and we must shape our habits and lifestyle according to our genetic heritage.

This knowledge has real practical value. It helps to know that a high cholesterol level isn't necessarily our fault. What's more, that high level warns us that we should have a complete evaluation of total blood fat and of the type of fat molecules involved. The evaluation is easy to do and can be performed by most doctors. The test results will help you know how rigid you must be with your diet and whether you should be on some type of medication that lowers the damaging type of cholesterol.

But what about cancer? Is cancer genetically caused? And if it is, what has gone wrong to cause it?

CANCER AND DAMAGED GENES

When we read a newspaper or book, we sometimes encounter an error that got by the proofreader. Perhaps it's a missing or mislpaced leter (just like the switched *l* and *p* in "mislpaced" and the missing *t* in "leter"). Given how easy it is to make a mistake in a short book like this one, think how many errors might be expected to creep into a letter code thirteen times longer than a thirty-two-volume encyclopedia!

What's amazing is a phenomenon described by Miroslave Radman and Robert Wagner in *Scientific American* (August, 1988). The two scientists point out that from generation to generation, and through countless cell divisions, the genetic heritage of living things is "scrupulously preserved" in the DNA. Since the human genetic code is some three billion letters long, even a one-in-a-million error would result in some 3,000 mistakes being made in a single duplication. Yet since you were conceived, your genomes have duplicated themselves about a *million billion* times—and very few, if any, mistakes in duplication have taken place!

But some mistakes do creep in. Microbiologists have discovered that even tiny mistakes can be devastating. For instance, the substitution of a single "letter" in the genetic code is the cause of diseases like hereditary sickle-cell anemia, Alzheimer's disease, cystic fibrosis, and several kinds of cancer.

Today cancer-causing genes have been given the name *oncogene,* a compound formed from *onco* (the root of the medical term meaning cancer) and *gene.* The discovery of oncogenes stunned the scientific community in the 1970s.

But another discovery astounded researchers even more: An oncogene in a cancer-causing virus was also found in healthy, normal cells! In fact, the cancer-causing gene was usually a normal, functioning part of a cell's DNA. Clearly, something had caused this normal gene to change into an oncogene and to prompt or contribute to malignant cell growth.

Suddenly new questions arose. What makes a normal, functioning gene turn into a potential killer? Which of the hundreds of thousands of genes within human beings are potential oncogenes? And, perhaps most significant, can our growing knowledge of cell biology help us defeat such genetically caused diseases? Scientists began dreaming about repairing defective genes and designing cancer-fighting agents that might function on the cellular level.

In 1989, researchers identified approximately fifty potentially cancer-causing genes in animals and humans, calling these genes *proto-oncogenes*. For instance, a single oncogene has been isolated from human bladder cancer cells. This gene, consisting of about 6,000 paired nucleotides (building blocks of amino acids and protein), differed in its normal form and its cancer-causing form by only *one* of the nucleotide pairs!

Think about that and you can begin to see why the capacity of the genome to duplicate itself with almost flawless accuracy is absolutely essential to our survival. Personally, I stand back in utter wonder at the wisdom of the Creator, who endowed living creatures with processes so absolutely, utterly amazing.

At present, research suggests that four events may transform proto-oncogenes into oncogenes. The proto-oncogene may be

1. damaged by some outside factor, such as radiation or contact with a carcinogen.
2. dislocated by movement from one DNA position to another.
3. activated by the movement of an unfamiliar gene next to it
4. amplified—that is, the cell's DNA may make too many copies of the same gene.

At present proto-oncogenes have been identified for only about twenty percent of the cancers in human beings. But intense research continues. Mounting evidence indicates that usually more than one oncogene is responsible for most cancers. For instance, colon cancer is now thought to involve some four to six genetic changes, and lung cancer may require from ten to fifteen genetic abnormalities. To sense what this means, visualize a slot machine with fifteen or twenty windows rather than the typical three or four. You pull the handle, the symbols within spin, and you get cancer only if all fifteen or twenty factors involved line up.

You can see how important it is to control elements of your lifestyle that are known to turn proto-oncogenes into oncogenes. For instance, we know that tobacco smoke is a major contributor to lung cancer. If you don't smoke—or if you quit—you may have closed enough windows on that biological slot machine to prevent lung cancer! It's the same with avoiding excess sun and staying away from alcohol. Giving up that suntan may prevent skin cancer. And avoiding alcohol may stop a fatal liver cancer before it gets started.

Again, if you wonder why some people who smoke escape lung cancer and some who don't smoke still get it, remember: every person's genetic heritage differs. Some may have genes without the potential flaws that promote a particular cancer, whatever their lifestyle. Others may have damaged genes that will line up in a cancer-causing pattern however carefully they live.

Modern discoveries about cancer remind us that you and I are responsible people. While our genetic heritage does have a dramatic effect on our physical health and well-being, genetics do not determine our future. We still have the freedom to *choose*. And in most cases, the choices we make *will* make a difference.

GENETIC CODES AND CANCER TREATMENT

The microbiologists' growing ability to "read" elements of a person's genetic code has already begun to have an impact on cancer treatment. For example, an experimental test developed by Robert Seeger of the Children's Hospital of Los Angeles and Garrett Brodeur of Washington University in St. Louis is capable of identifying multiple copies of a mutated gene in the tumor cells of *neuroblastoma,* a rare childhood cancer. Doctors recently surgically removed such a tumor in an eighteen-month-old girl. But they wondered whether or not she also should receive a more painful follow-up treatment. Based on analysis of the cancer gene, the toddler was given chemotherapy, whole-body radiation, and a bone-marrow transplant. And there, in the bone marrow, Seeger found tiny new tumors! Gene analysis had correctly indicated a need for further treatment—treatment that most likely saved a little girl's life.

Gene analysis not only helps doctors determine which patients should have further treatment after surgery, but soon it also will identify people who have inherited defective oncogenes. This capacity will enable the medical community to prevent cancer in a number of ways: we can warn people with defective oncogenes to stay away from carcinogens that may trigger a cancer outbreak, and we can monitor people who are most susceptible to cancer, enabling us to identify and treat a cancer in its early stages, when a total cure is much more probable.

Still, what is most exciting is that the discoveries we are making today about the inner workings of the cell hold the promise of actually eradicating cancer in the future! In the next chapter, I explain more about that.

9

THE BODY'S DEFENSES

The last chapter explained how recent advances in microbiology have led to many discoveries about the causes of cancer. These same advances have helped us understand more fully the complex interactions of our body's immune system—that built-in, natural defense system that fights enemies of good health like bacteria, viruses—and cancers. But how?

Medical research is making two spectacular scientific breakthroughs: we've begun to understand what's going on in our body's immune system, and we've begun to glimpse ways in which that understanding can help us conquer cancer.

This chapter will try to help you understand the terminology used to describe the dynamics of your immune system. When you understand some of the basic concepts outlined in this chapter, you will be better able to follow the cancer-research progress reported in articles and news reports.

THE BODY'S DEFENSES

HOW YOUR IMMUNE SYSTEM WORKS

The immune system is composed of cells, most of which are highly specialized white blood cells that have the ability to move beyond our blood vessels and patrol between tissue cells. We can liken these white blood cells to a large police force, always on guard, seeking any indication of invaders who break in and threaten the host—you.

Your body activates literally trillions of these specialized cells at all times. In fact, the normal white-cell count in a single drop of blood the size of a pinhead is 4,000 to 5,000! As the average person has about six quarts of blood, you can see how vast an army of protective cells is involved in your defense.

White blood cells are divided into two general classes: a *granulocyte* has many different lobes in its nucleus; a *monocyte* has a single, oval nucleus. We're particularly interested in the monocyte, which is represented by *macrophages* (sometimes called *phagocytes*) and the *lymphocytes*.

Macrophages

Macrophages are huge, lumbering cells, whose duty is to clean up the debris left after the body battles an infection or an invader. The macrophage does this by encircling the debris and consuming it. In fact, the macrophage will surround anything that doesn't belong in the body—including cancer cells! The problem is that our bodies don't produce enough macrophages to keep pace with something like cancer.

You can understand why when you consider how rapidly some cancer cells multiply. Like other cells in the body, cancer cells duplicate themselves by doubling. One cell becomes two, two become four, four become eight, and so on. The average length of time it takes for all the cells in a tumor to duplicate themselves has been called the doubling time. For instance, by the time a cancerous mass in the breast can be felt, it's about the size of a pea. It has gone through at least thirty reduplications and will contain over a billion cells! Depending on the kind of cancer, the doubling time for breast cancers can be as little as six days or as long as a year and a half. Given the quickest rate, over a billion cancer cells will be generated in six months in a single, tiny breast tumor. It's no wonder that the macrophage cells in the body, busy fighting other invaders as well as cancer, simply can't keep up.

Lymphocytes

Lymphocytes, the chief cells in the immune system, make up about forty percent of all white blood cells. Lymphocytes are formed in the bone marrow of the sternum, ribs, vertebrae, pelvis, legs, and arms.

When a cancerous cell is discovered, the lymphocyte kills it and takes a fragment of its DNA molecule. The lymphocyte then rushes through the blood vessels and tissues and does two things: it spreads chemical warnings to identify the invader, and it specifies the chemical agent to be used in fighting the enemy.

In the 1940s and 1950s, we knew that the lymphocyte was part of the immune system and that such cells congregated in the lymph nodes. We knew the cell had something to do with acute infections because then the lymph glands would swell and become tender. But in the 1970s, an information explosion raised the awareness of the importance of the lymphocyte. Further research indicates that this cell might provide the key to overcoming not only cancer, but also AIDS. For with the development of the electron microscope, we've been able both to distinguish types of lymphocytes and also to chart their role in defending the body.

Two critical types of lymphocytes have been labeled *T* cells and *B* cells. T cells have been called the "floating brain" of the defense system, for they diagnose and develop strategies to battle against invaders. These cells patrol the body, and when an enemy—bacteria, virus, or cancer cell—is discovered, T cells fire a chemical called a *lymphokine*, which kills the enemy. The T cells then take a portion of the enemy and race through the body, alerting the immune system and advising what biological weapon to use in the counterattack. It's no wonder that the T cell has earned the nickname "Killer Cell." Even more amazing, the T cell has the ability to identify 18 *million* different enemies, and the ability to defend against them by selecting *and creating* the particular lymphokine the situation demands! Thus the T cell acts as spy, watchman, soldier, and general in the battle against foreign invaders.

The impact of this discovery is seen in the much-publicized attempts to duplicate the lymphokines that are produced by the body's own defense system. So far the chief lymphokines used today against cancers are *interferon* and *interleukin,* neither of which has proven to be the definitive answer against cancer, as some had optimistically predicted. Yet in the future, researchers expect to identify the body's naturally produced cancer-killing substances and then duplicate those substances to defeat specific cancers. These treatments may be able to replace traumatic treatments like radiation and chemotherapy.

The second significant kind of lymphocyte is the B cell, a warrior programmed by the T cell to produce specific antibodies and antitoxins. The T cell also triggers the body to produce more B cells, and even can transform B cells into T cells when a threat to the body requires. In this role, the T cell is referred to as the "Helper Cell." When the battle is over, the

T cells order the B cells to retreat—to quit producing. In this role, the T cell is called the "Suppressor Cell."

The B cell itself is a specialized lymphocyte larger than the T cell. B cells live only a few days, while the smaller T cells may live for months or years. While the B cells are "cannon fodder," soldiers sent to fight and die, the T cell is the general, living on to direct the body's battle.

The B cell matures into a plasma cell, which produces antibodies and immune globulin. The antibodies the B cell produces are specifically designed by the T cell to attack the protein of the invader cell. In the struggle against cancer, these antibodies not only fight present tumors, but antibodies remain in the blood to resist a relapse. In fact, after the battle is won, T cells and B cells together form memory cells that record the struggle and guard against the defeated enemy's return!

This whole process is complicated, I know. It may even seem confusing the first time you read this through. Actually, it's far more complicated than I've described. But what I want you to grasp is that an amazing and effective biological defense system already exists within your body.

That defense system continues to fight every kind of disease and illness, including fighting the cancer cells that are present even in healthy people. What's more, as we are beginning to understand more about how this defense system works, we've come across clues to new ways to fight cancer. As we learn more, we'll almost certainly be able to develop better and better cancer-fighting tools.

In the future you'll be reading about custom-made cancer antibodies, created by microbiologists, that will lead to the defeat of every malignancy! And, beyond that, there is the prospect of vaccines that may make cancer as rare in the future as polio is today!

THE BODY'S DEFENSES

BOLSTERING YOUR IMMUNE SYSTEM

The next chapter will describe more prospects for future cancer treatments. Now, though, I want to mention something that is still a mystery. Your *attitude* can either help or hinder your immune system's fight against cancer. We don't understand completely why this is true, but more and more evidence indicates that your attitude plays a critical role.

Let me illustrate by telling you about Emil, a successful real-estate broker and investor. Emil was a popular community leader, a man people liked to be around. He always had a cheery greeting, an infectious smile, and a good story to tell. I frequently associated with Emil on different hospital boards and in various community affairs. I liked working with him.

Then it happened. One morning, plastered all over the front page of our newspaper, was a story of Emil's indictment for fraud. This was especially hard because Emil had always prided himself on his honesty and integrity. No one could believe it, and no one wanted to believe it. I trusted him before the story hit the newspaper, and I trusted him after it appeared.

But somehow it seemed to Emil that everything he had lived for had collapsed around him. After the indictment, Emil just seemed to disappear. He wasn't seen on the street or in his usual meeting places for breakfast. He stopped attending his service clubs. It was obvious that he was hurting badly. This charge against him was particularly painful because he had always gone the extra mile to be fair.

Not long afterward I saw him in my office—as a patient. His smile was gone, and he told no stories. He was nauseated and couldn't sleep. He began to suffer from headaches and dizzy spells. Soon he developed shingles and didn't do well at all. His wife, a nervous person anyway, was beside herself.

She could do nothing to cheer him up. He was broken in spirit, and somehow this had led to a physical as well as emotional breakdown.

I've seen this all too often during my years in medical practice. Somehow emotional trauma, anxiety, disappointments, or losses seem to inhibit the body's natural defenses. In extreme cases like Emil's, it may even cause the defenses to malfunction or collapse.

The months went by, and Emil continued to suffer emotionally and physically. Finally it was time for the trial, and again he was front-page news. But this time Emil was vindicated. He was acquitted of all charges.

But Emil's health did not change. The smearing of his reputation so wounded him that he was unable to take his old place in the community. After a few months he retired and moved away.

I've seen Emil several times since then, and I'm happy to report that he's slowly regaining his health. But it was obvious that the false accusations took their toll, and that he could maintain his equilibrium only by avoiding the area that had caused him all his pain.

I share that story because it illustrates two things you need to understand. First, your attitude during treatment for cancer or for any other disease can have an impact on your recovery. If you let yourself slide into despair, if you refuse to work through anger, if you simply give up, your immune system will function less effectively. On the other hand, if you are able to maintain a positive attitude, to accept and then deal positively with your disease, the functioning of your immune system will be enhanced.

Yes, I know you'll have down times. We all do. But I'm speaking here of overall attitude, of your general approach to coping with your disease.

In the last ten years much has been made of the interrelationship of attitude and health. Doctors have noted that the more optimistic their patients are, the more efficiently their immune systems function, and the healthier and better they feel. On the other hand, pessimistic patients—those who feel depressed, worried, sensitive, frightened—tend to feel much worse than the optimistic patients.

Then Norman Cousins and his book *Anatomy of an Illness* stimulated interest in somehow *measuring* whatever it was that made the one class of patients do better. From the University of South Florida, Dr. Nicholas Hall has contributed some interesting findings that have helped to measure factors that make a difference. But this is just the beginning of a breakthrough in a very important phase of medicine. Attitude is a very powerful force. It not only causes subjective changes, it also influences the operation of various bodily systems. The person who is constantly anxious and pessimistic subjects his or her bodily systems to stress which will, in one way or another, result in a breakdown.

Chapters 6 and 7 of this book suggest ways to overcome that sense of hopelessness and powerlessness that often strike cancer patients. And my cancer diary in Part III of this book shares some of the feelings and experiences that I had as I fought my own battle with cancer. I've included meditative readings that may help keep your attitude positive and hopeful. They're there because I know how important attitude is in your struggle with this disease. They're there because I want to nurture your inner person as well as give you solid medical reasons for hope in your battle to conquer cancer.

But the second reason I include Emil's story is to emphasize the fact that *a positive attitude isn't everything.* Too many books offer false hope. Too many talk show guests have said that if you only stay upbeat and positive, your body will heal itself. I have no patience with those who make the rounds of talk shows suggesting you treat cancer with a smile!

After all, you wouldn't treat a broken leg with laughter. You would get the bone set. You wouldn't expect a positive attitude to reduce the level of cholesterol in your blood. You would change your diet, and, if necessary, you would take medication to reduce the chance of heart attack. Why in the world, then, would anyone expect to cure malignancies through a positive attitude?

Please don't buy into that "eat-our-diet-and-think-positively" school of cancer therapy. There's a word for most people who rely on that. The word is, *statistic.*

Certainly I want you to maintain a positive attitude. It's a lot better for your immune system than those negative attitudes that depress the system. But remember that a positive attitude is not by itself going to produce a cure. A cure comes through medical treatment and the functioning of a complex immune system that automatically, without any conscious effort on your part, struggles against malignant cells.

And what a relief this should be. Think what a burden it would be if I told you fighting cancer depended solely on your attitude. Think how you would feel if your cancer got worse. Not only would you face death, but you also would feel guilty because somehow you failed!

I've run into similar thinking with some of my religious patients, who assume that God will heal only if they have enough faith. As a Christian, I believe that God can and does heal. But I also believe that God has enabled us to develop wonderful medical treatments for fighting our diseases. Why assume that God is involved in a person's battle with cancer only if he performs a miracle? To me, the real miracle is the amazing immune system the Creator designed, a system that so effectively guards us as well as heals. My task as a Christian physician is to use every tool God has put at my disposal—including prayer, medical treatments, and modern drugs—to promote healing. Your privilege as a Christian patient is not to reject medical help, but to thank God for providing it!

Today our knowledge of DNA and the immune system is exploding. More information is coming in constantly, from all over the world. In addition to all the money spent by government agencies in cancer research, more millions are being invested by drug companies, eager to bring profitable anticancer drugs on the market. In one recent period, the government devoted $24 million to genetic research, and pharmaceutical companies poured $200 million into the search for new genetic agents for fighting cancer. Whatever the motive of those paying for the research, one thing is excitingly clear: What we know now points the way to even more effective cancer-fighting tools—tools that will be developed in the near future, tools you'll soon be reading about in your daily newspaper, tools I'll tell you about in the next chapter.

10

DEVELOPMENTS TO WATCH

The medical discoveries relating to oncogenes and the immune system have led to exciting developments in our battle against cancer. A host of new weapons are being developed. Some weapons have already been reported in the popular media, and a flood of articles and features are sure to follow. This chapter will give you a brief overview to help you understand the most promising developments that you'll read and hear about.

GENE SPLICING

The concept of splicing is similar to the ancient art of grafting. Farmers take branches from cultivated fruit trees and graft them (attach the new branch to a cut on the old trunk or branch) into wild trees whose fruit is small or bitter. When the graft takes, the branches of the cultivated fruit trees grow and produce larger, sweeter fruit.

Gene splicing involves grafting a desirable protein into a bacteria so that when the bacteria multiplies, the desirable protein is also duplicated.

Earlier I explained how T-cell lymphocytes in our bodies analyze a cancer and devise a cancer-killing lymphokine (chemical weapon) to use against it. Each lymphokine is a specially designed chemical, intended to attack just one enemy. In the case of cancer, these chemicals are called *cytokines*.

Recently scientists have been able to harvest some of these anticancer lymphokines. They have identified specific anti-cancer proteins, and by gene splicing have introduced them into certain easily controlled bacteria. The process produces much more of the specific anticancer substance, which is then injected into a cancer victim to help him or her fight the disease.

MONOCLONAL ANTIBODIES

We've all seen those detective movies in which a tiny transmitter is planted with the ransom money so that the police can follow the cash to the criminals. If we think of the cancer as a transmitter, we can understand monoclonal antibodies as unique medical creations that "hone in" on the cancer cells.

Creating a monoclonal antibody is a very complicated process. Several immune-system compounds extracted from blood cells and several live tumor cells are injected into a mouse, which produces *antibodies* to fight the injected material. The mouse's spleen is removed, and the cells that produced these antibodies are removed and fused with

167

CONQUERING CANCER

GENE SPLICING

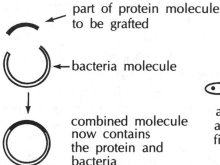
part of protein molecule to be grafted

bacteria molecule

combined molecule now contains the protein and bacteria

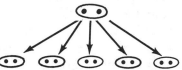
a new molecule multiplies and produces more cancer-fighting proteins

This diagram, a modification of a diagram found in the March 19, 1988, issue of the *Journal of the American Medical Association,* shows how the splicing is done.

---

cancerous cells from another mouse. These cells are then duplicated (cloned). The result of this process is a cell that seeks out and bonds with specific proteins on the surface of a living cancer cell in the cancer patient.

At the moment, monoclonal antibodies' greatest value is diagnostic, for they locate and identify cancers very early, when they are most vulnerable. But researchers are working hard to turn monoclonals into cancer fighters.

In London's Imperial Cancer Research Fund, doctors used monoclonals to carry tiny beads of iron oxide to cancer cells. They then used magnets in an attempt to "pull" the cancer cells out of bone marrow! This treatment is currently used at the University of Florida and UCLA. Duke University plans to try this method on patients with rapidly growing breast cancers.

An article in the *Journal of the American Medical Association*

(January 12, 1990) suggests directing monoclonals against critical structures on the cancer cell's surface. Cell membranes are made up of various proteins that have special functions. Some proteins function as *receptors*. Like the doors in a warehouse, these receptors provide an entrance through which needed foods from the bloodstream can be absorbed. It may be possible to design monoclonals that not only seek out cancer cells but also find a specific receptor and command it to "open the door!" If researchers are successful in turning monoclonals into carriers of radioactive isotopes, toxins, and drugs, a monoclonal might not only find the receptor and tell it to open the door, but then it might go through the open door and deliver a killing poison directly into the heart of the cancer cell!

GENETIC ENGINEERING

Genetic engineering uses amazing new technologies to modify and repair the genes of a living person. It holds out the possibility of eradicating not only cancer but also many other genetically caused diseases.

Earlier I noted that microbiologists have been able to locate cancer-causing genes, called oncogenes. But this is not all that scientists can do with genes. Through the use of two machines, the *protein sequenator* and the *protein synthesizer,* they now can actually "read" the chemical components of the genes and synthesize them.

Protein Sequenator

To understand the protein sequenator, imagine you have a pair of scissors in one hand and a long chain of fine metallic links in the other hand. You take your scissors, clip off just one link, examine it, and jot down what it's made of—silver or brass or gold or tin or whatever. Snip by snip, you remove the links of the chain, each time recording the metal. When every link has been removed, your notebook contains a string of notations, like "tin, tin, silver, gold, platinum, tin, gold, silver, silver" and so on.

You now know exactly how that chain was made, and if you want to, you can duplicate that chain simply by stringing links of the correct metal in order. What's more, if you happen to have a *faulty* chain—one that left out the silver link that is third in the sequence—you might even fix that chain by adding the missing silver link.

The protein sequenator works in a similar way: it uses chemical scissors to clip off one link of a linear protein chain that is found in our genes. The link, made up of an amino acid, is clipped off, identified, and its position on the chain recorded. In this way the "code" of an antibody, or of our genes and chromosomes themselves, can be "read."

Protein Synthesizer

Once the protein sequenator reads the code of a DNA fragment, cancer antibody, or gene, the protein synthesizer comes into play. This device synthesizes proteins by starting at one end and adding the appropriate amino acid in sequence to the growing chain! This ability to synthesize proteins means that we can *artificially* generate those fragments of larger molecules that fight cancer, use them to immunize rabbits or mice, and in time very likely create vaccines that may make a human being immune to cancer!

It's hard to grasp how rapid our progress in learning to understand and manipulate the immune system and DNA has been. Today a commercial version of a machine developed at California Institute of Technology is able to synthesize DNA fragments 180 nucleotides long, at the rate of one nucleotide every fourteen minutes. In nine hours, with one part-time assistant, a small gene can be synthesized. If this seems slow, consider the work of Har Gobind Khorana at the University of Wisconsin in the 1970s. Working with twenty-five post-doctoral fellows, it took Dr. Khorana *six years* to do the same thing!

With more genes with which to work in the laboratory, researchers will be able to use many more anticancer amino acids and proteins and will be able to make them more specific for individual patients. The potential of this approach to disease is limitless. Already, human insulin is harvested and used, eliminating the drawbacks of the old method. Vaccines and antiviral drugs will be made. Just think of the possibility of vaccinating against breast cancer and virtually eliminating the disease, just as we did with polio. And then, if by chance, a woman develops a cancer, we can take a sample of the tumor, culture it, and produce volumes of a specific anticancer drug to eradicate the cancer. Scientists will be able to do this with many kinds of cancer, eliminating them one by one.

For many tumors, like the one my brother Karl had, the time is here. My own tumor was eradicated as recently as fifteen years ago. Technology saved my life. The discoveries will come one by one, but they will come increasingly faster.

Gene Manipulation

Our new tools have made it possible to analyze genes, to determine absent or excess elements in oncogenes, and possibly even to change living cells to prevent the development of cancer. For instance, the gene that gives bacteria the ability to resist the antibiotic neomycin was isolated and put into a crippled virus. These were multiplied in test tubes, with interleukin-2, and some 200 billion of these cells were injected into each patient. These manipulated cells lived on in

171

the blood stream for up to half a year, and biopsies performed over two months after injection showed that the cells had penetrated the tumors—and were reproducing bacterial protein.

Soon researchers will insert the gene that makes tumor necrosis factor, a powerful cancer killer, into human blood cells. This will increase the production of this protein and intensify the body's attack on a tumor.

But there's even more potential here. Microbiologists Webster Cavenee and Raymond White discovered gene markers on chromosome 13 that enabled them to identify a gene which, when damaged, caused a cancer of the retina of the eye. They then "coaxed" samples of the gene to produce the protein that, when missing, causes the cancer. This may lead to a new class of cancer therapy: a therapy in which, rather than killing tumor cells, genetic engineers introduce missing proteins that may cause damaged cells to act like normal ones!

THE HUMAN GENOME PROJECT

Another promising cancer-fighting approach is the human genome project. Earlier I noted that the DNA in human beings contains some 3 billion molecules. I said that if a letter were assigned to each of these molecules, and each letter were printed in sequence as it lies along the DNA strand, the code of a single human being would fill over thirteen sets of the thirty-two volume *Encyclopedia Britannica*. The total of that material, genes, chromosomes, and other DNA is called the "genome."

In the past ten years, genes or genetic markers for over 300 disorders have been found. But to master the promising new techniques just now emerging, we need a much more accurate knowledge of the sequence and significance of *all* material in the human genome. In response to that need, interested scientists launched the Human Genome Project in January 1989. This group intends to "map" the entire human DNA molecule, identifying each of the 3 billion chemical particles, in sequence. For the next fifteen years, thousands of researchers will be involved, at costs exceeding $3 billion. But the result will be a map that will enable researchers to associate genes not only with cancers but also with scores of other genetically caused diseases. The map will help clinicians pinpoint genetic abnormalities and develop therapies to repair or negate them!

Within the next few years we can expect a steady flow of new diagnostic tests, therapies, and technologies to be generated by the project. Let me give one illustration. Researchers at the National Cancer Institute in Maryland have identified special T lymphocytes that can actually infiltrate (enter) tumors. This is important, because melanomas are normally so dense that most mobile cells can't enter them. Yet T lymphocytes seek out these tumors and penetrate them. So the next step will be to remove the T lymphocytes from cancer patients, splice in a gene that produces a cancer-killing substance, and return them to the body to carry this substance into the heart of the tumor itself! While many problems need to be solved before such techniques are in common use, the prospect for tomorrow is extremely bright.

INTERFERON RESEARCH

Interferons are a group of natural body proteins that "interfere" with a cancer cell's ability to reproduce. Interferons were originally identified as antiviral (anti-virus) agents and later found to have some anticancer value. In the late

1970s and early 1980s, the American Cancer Society provided massive support for clinical trials to test this activity in humans.

Interferons have not proven to be the miracle cure for cancer, as people in the early 1980s had hoped. But interferons have had a significant success rate in treating certain conditions. For instance, ninety percent of people with hairy-cell leukemia, a rare but once invariably fatal cancer, are cured by treatments of alpha-interferon. In May 1986, alpha-interferon became the first of the new cancer drugs to be approved by the Food and Drug Administration.

One present drawback with interferon is that it's effective only in high doses, and massive doses have highly toxic side effects. Even so, the lifesaving impact of alpha-interferon on hairy-cell leukemia and significant results in treating other cancers suggest that as we learn more about cell biology, interferons will have a role in our final victory.

CARCINOGENESIS RESEARCH

The term *carcinogenesis* is a compound formed from the two roots *carcino* (related to cancer) and *genesis* (origin). Thus the term identifies research in the origins of cancer.

In an earlier chapter I introduced you to oncogenes and proto-oncogenes. Carcinogenesis research attempts to answer questions about these cancer-causing and potentially cancer-causing genes.

If we use an analogy, proto-oncogenes and oncogenes are like light switches. Electricity is always flowing through a house's wiring, but only if we turn the light switch on will a particular lamp light up. If we view cancer as something that is similarly "switched on," we can pose a number of important questions for research to answer. For instance, which cells serve as switches in early cancer development? Which cells serve as switches to turn cancer on later in life? What specifically turns these switches on? And, can they be programmed to stay switched off?

We already have evidence that certain viruses cause cancer in humans, perhaps by activating proto-oncogenes. And we have also found a normal gene that appears *to suppress* the development of cancer. For instance, one discovery indicates that colon cancer develops over the course of years through a series of genetic changes or mutations that really are like turning on a set of switches that promote growth, while turning off others that retard growth.

This whole field is very new, made public in 1989 when two American physicians who discovered oncogenes were awarded a Nobel prize. Once the Human Genome Project enables us to isolate more oncogenes, we can use already existing biological tools to analyze their specific structure. In an article appearing in the 1989 issue of *Surgery, Gynecology & Obstetrics,* Michael A. Skinner and J. Dirk Iglehart say, "As more knowledge accumulates regarding the exact mechanisms through which the proteins encoded by oncogenes affect these carcinomas and others, it may become possible to design pharmacological agents rationally to hinder their growth selectively." In plainer English, they anticipate the creation of specific drugs that will stop the growth of potentially cancerous cells, even before the cells become malignant!

DIFFERENTIATION MODIFIERS

Differentiation modifiers are growth factors that regulate and control the multiplication of cells. When tumors develop, the cancerous cells have somehow escaped these normal controls. Some growth factors, as well as some inhibitors that change the effect of these factors, have been identified. What may lie ahead, as these complex processes are better understood, is that differentiation modifiers may be injected to instruct cancerous cells to stop reproducing and to lead them back to their originally intended function in the body.

Even today some growth factors that regulate proliferation of blood cells are in clinical trials. These growth factors may be used to stimulate the ability of bone marrow to produce white-blood-cell defenses against infections related to immunodeficiency disorders.

DRUG DEVELOPMENT

In addition to the many doorways opened to cancer researchers by microbiological advances, work is also being done to develop new anticancer drugs. This is important because most anticancer drugs now in use are poisonous not only to the cancer cells but also to the normal ones. The search continues for drugs that will be less harmful to normal cells and more specifically targeted to tumors.

A wide variety of anticancer drugs is also needed because the body develops its own resistance to them. Using a variety of different drugs makes it less likely that resistance will develop and more likely that the tumor will be eliminated.

Even *Business Week,* in its June 26, 1989, issue, noted that one new family of anticancer drugs is being tested by the UpJohn pharmaceutical company. This synthetic version of a toxic cell killer was almost discarded until UpJohn chemists separated the cancer-killing element from the parts that harm normal cells. UpJohn reports that these compounds attach to the DNA of cancerous cells and prevent them from reproducing.

When we put the ongoing research projects into perspective and see the amazing strides made in the past ten years and even five years, we have many reasons to be optimistic. We will conquer cancer. And in the next few years, you'll be reading more about the treatment types I've introduced you to in this chapter. Because of the advances already made, as well as those just around the corner, a person with cancer today has a far more realistic basis for hope than at any other time in history!

A FINAL REMINDER

When you read about the new discoveries in cancer research, remember that the treatments reported in popular journals are experimental. Just like the treatments I've reviewed in this chapter, they hold great promise, but they are neither available to everyone—nor perfected.

I'm confident that current genetics research will lead to the total conquest of cancer. But at the moment, these techniques are experimental. Don't let an article in a popular magazine lead you to believe that an experimental treatment has become standard.

And be careful in choosing your doctor. You may not want to become a guinea pig for a theoretically promising but not yet practically proven cancer treatment.

In the meantime, keep the faith.

As you or your loved one struggle with cancer, remember that the longer you can hang on, the more likely you will find a total cure.

PART III

A Cancer Diary

A CANCER DIARY

For years I've observed the emotions of my patients as they fought cancer. Then I had to face cancer myself. I experienced the uncertainties and the setbacks. I searched for comfort and fought to maintain hope. I came to know intimately the emotional reactions I had observed in others.

In this section I identify twelve of the most common emotional and psychological states a cancer sufferer is likely to experience: disbelief, isolation, uncertainty, resignation, courage, searching, comfort, growing confidence, stretching, setting goals, sensitivity, and thankfulness. I share some of my own feelings about each state and include several readings for thought and meditation. My goal is not only to help you better understand your own feelings but also to share insights that may strengthen you. The readings are brief and include poetry, epigrammatic reflections on the theme, Scripture, medical bulletins, and even practical suggestions. You may want simply to skim through this section at first. Then, as you find yourself in one of the emotional or psychological states I describe, return and meditate on a favorite reading or two.

You may find it helpful to start your own cancer diary. You won't always feel up to writing in it. That's okay. Come back to it when you do. Also clip out and include readings that help you deal with your feelings and maintain hope.

Remember: Whatever you experience, you're not alone.

Others have passed this way before. Others have found the strength that you will discover too—strength to face the future with courage and hope.

DISBELIEF

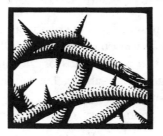

"I feel numb and confused. There must be some mistake. This can't possibly be! I mean, I feel so good. I have no pain."

How hard we try to avoid reality. Knowing you have cancer is a time of confusion, mixed with helplessness. This is a time when, as a doctor, I'm very careful with what I say. I share the diagnosis very simply, without too much detail. I give time for questions. It's really time for me to turn into a good listener. For many, this first stage doesn't go away quickly. Patients have told me how lost they felt; how out of step with society.

"I understand now. I'm a doctor, but I can't practice any longer. I'm a doctor/patient, no longer quite who I was, uncertain just who I will become."

I cannot find my way: there is no star
In all the shrouded heavens anywhere;
And there is not a whisper in the air

CONQUERING CANCER

Of any living voice but one so far
That I can hear it only as a bar
Of lost, imperial music, played when fair
And angel fingers wove, and unaware,
Dead leaves to garlands where no roses are.

No, there is not a glimmer, nor a call,
For one that welcomes, welcomes when he fears,
The black and awful chaos of the night;
For through it all—above, beyond it all—
I know the far-sent message of the years,
I feel the coming glory of the Light.

—Edwin Arlington Robinson
"Credo"

There are over 6 million Americans today who have a history of cancer, 3 million of them diagnosed five or more years ago. Most of these 3 million can be considered cured, while others still have evidence of cancer. By "cured" it is meant that a patient has no evidence of the disease and has the same life expectancy as a person who never had cancer.

—*Cancer Facts and Figures 1990*
The American Cancer Society

The only courage that matters is the kind that gets you from one moment to the next.

—Mignon McLaughlin

DISBELIEF

Guilt is a persistent and unwelcome companion of many cancer patients. Nagging, half-formed questions dog our heels and nip at the nighttime thoughts of our loved ones.

Among the pack that follows us is, "What did I do to cause my disease?" "I shouldn't be doing this to my family." And, "It isn't fair that others are well while I'm not."

Among those nipping at our loved ones are, "What did I do to cause his sickness?" "Why do I resent all my new responsibilities? It's not his fault, and I'm really sorry for him." And, "I'm scared. What will happen to us if he dies?"

All we have to throw at these feelings to drive them away is the truth. No one is to blame. My cancer is a fact of life that we have to learn to deal with.

What's more, we can. And we will.

The LORD is my shepherd, I shall not be in want.
 He makes me lie down in green pastures,
he leads me beside quiet waters,
 he restores my soul.
He guides me in paths of righteousness
 for his name's sake.
Even though I walk
 through the valley of the shadow of death,
I will fear no evil,
 for you are with me;
your rod and your staff,
 they comfort me.

You prepare a table before me
   in the presence of my enemies.
You anoint my head with oil;
   my cup overflows.
Surely goodness and love will follow me
   all the days of my life,
and I will dwell in the house of the LORD
   forever.

               —Psalm 23

It was during the test when we discovered my cancer. The X rays were complete, and John Maxwell and I were alone in the viewing room. During our discussion, another doctor walked in and saw the films. His remark was, "I'm sure glad those aren't my X rays."

To which I answered, "You don't have to worry any, Ed. Those are mine."

We all started to laugh nervously, and we've discussed that incident many times since. Ed said he wished he could have found an eject button so he could have disappeared. But I didn't give him that luxury. In fact, it broke the tension, and I felt a lot better for the moment. Really, during my cancer I never felt so much love in my life, not only from my family but also from the entire hospital staff and from friends I hadn't heard from for years. It's just amazing how news like that travels.

To be courageous requires no exceptional qualifications, no magic formula, no special combination of time, place and circumstance. It is an opportunity that sooner or later is presented to us all.

—John F. Kennedy

Prayer

Lord, guide me through this rushing stream of swirling thoughts and fears, to the calmer waters that must flow just beyond.

ISOLATION

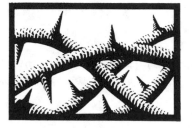

"I don't want to see anyone these days except my family. Yes, and my partner, who has always been close to me. For some reason I feel more secure alone. Small talk bothers me. I don't want to discuss my problem with well-meaning friends, and it's painful to be exposed to well-wishers. I want a place where no one can find me, not even by telephone. I just want to go to sleep and not be bothered. I can't concentrate, even on reading or watching television. It seems as if my brain is in neutral."

Looking back, I realized many of my patients have had this reaction. I understood that I could easily slip into depression. The world had come to a temporary halt. What helped me was getting ready for the diagnostic tests and treatment. I stayed so busy that I didn't have time to feel sorry for myself.

We haven't got time to feel sorry for ourselves just now. We've got a great team of doctors. We've got their instructions to follow. We've got gallons of apple juice to drink and cleansing laxatives to take. We have to get ready for our surgery or radiation or chemotherapy. We can't withdraw. We have treatments to take. We've got to get up, to keep on—on our way to victory.

I took my "death wish" to the cemetery today. And there, amid granite grave markers and plastic flowers, was death.

Weeping willows drooped and rustled in gentle wind— they were alive. Frogs made lively leaps into a deathless "man made" pond. Both willows and amphibians lived their fragile lives unaware that death was near on every side.

I felt alone and out of place.

I had just said, "My life is over!" And so it seemed at the moment. Faced with deadly sickness in my soul and spirit, I was sure I could not go on living another day. My world seemed on the verge of utter collapse. All I had worked for was about to slip through my defeat-numbed fingers.

The stark and dreadful reality of my inner sickness mingled with the melody of a worship song coming from somewhere inside me—mocking my true emptiness and faithlessness with a dreadful irony. Hope—dashed again and again by my "uncontrollable" anger and sinful outbursts—seemed dead and gone.

"There is no hope!" I had bitterly sobbed.

All whose buried earthly tents that lie around me now, are in the process of being forgotten. If, like me, any of them ever hoped that his death would emphasize his existence, or would underscore his cries for help, or would gain him sympathy, concern, or notice he felt he lacked in life, if somewhere he is conscious, he now knows that death has accomplished none of these things! It may have come as a shock, a deep grief, or a relief to the living left to deal with his memory. But it was not emphasis, nor the filling of some lack. Death was just . . . the end. The beginning of the process of being forgotten. As years go by, both the pain and joy in knowing "our dear departed" will be enhazed in the blurry banks of increasingly distant memory. Soon, no one will even mention his name.

Is that good or bad? Is that what I have been wishing for? Does my heart really desire the inevitable anonymity of the "departed"?

—Bob Girard
Written in a cemetery near
Scottsdale, Arizona, in 1978
from *My Weakness: His Strength*

Listen to my prayer, O God,
   do not ignore my plea;
   hear me and answer me.
My thoughts trouble me and I am distraught
   at the voice of the enemy,
   at the stares of the wicked;
for they bring down suffering upon me
   and revile me in their anger.

My heart is in anguish within me;
   the terrors of death assail me.
Fear and trembling have beset me;
   horror has overwhelmed me.
I said, "Oh, that I had the wings of a dove!
   I would fly away and be at rest—
I would flee far away

and stay in the desert;
I would hurry to my place of shelter,
far from the tempest and storm."

But I call to God,
and the LORD saves me.
Evening, morning and noon
I cry out in distress,
and he hears my voice.
He ransoms me unharmed
from the battle waged against me,
even though many oppose me.

Cast your cares on the LORD
and he will sustain you;
he will never let the righteous fall.
As for me, I trust in you.

—David
from Psalm 55

Being alone can be truly therapeutic. I'm convinced that everyone must have some time alone. This accomplishes several things. It gives us time for prioritizing our values. Things that seem important in a routine world take on a different definition and importance when we stand back and look at the whole picture. It's so easy to get locked into a set routine or a pattern which in the final analysis isn't that important. The first reaction most people have is that they don't have time to be alone. That just isn't true. I have found that the best time is the first thing in the morning, just after getting up. It's quiet, with no sounds of television or radio. Fifteen minutes alone sets the tone for the whole day.

What do you do during that time? You get in touch with yourself, and you get in touch with God. You talk to him, you thank him. You pray for yourself and others. This is time for deep spiritual relationships, for meditation and renewal of your commitment. And you start the day cleansed and refreshed.

Having time alone, and being alone, are different things. When you feel a need for others, when you want to hear a friendly voice or share your uncertainty, you *can* find people who care.

Hospitals often set up group and individual counseling sessions for cancer outpatients who want and need emotional support. Your doctor can probably put you in touch with such a group in your community. Or you may turn to the "Where to Find Help" section in the back of the book.

One psychologist recently observed, "Blessed are the insensitive slobs." What he meant was, how good it would be if we couldn't be hurt. How many marriages would then hold together, and how many parents and children would find anger and pain gone away. If we were insensitive, how much easier it would be to do the right thing, never worrying about the possibility of rejection or ridicule from others.

Of course, God has a better idea. As usual, his approach is to cause us to become increasingly tender. With that tenderness, he provides us with his own matchless willingness to forgive. We are all sure to hurt and to be hurt. But when we

192

forgive, and accept forgiveness, we make the wonderful discovery that it is the healing and not the absence of hurts that binds us closer to others, and to God.

Prayer

Lord, melt the ice of the isolation that shock and fear have frozen tight around me. Thaw my heart with love—the love of others, and your own.

Uncertainty

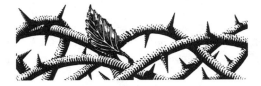

"I've gradually emerged into the realization that, at least for the present, I'm going to live. But I have no idea what the future holds. Still, I may as well settle into my life, even though it is studded with doubt. But even in the midst of the doubt, I also feel a ray of hope.

"My doctors are so supportive. They radiate hope, but not unreasonable hope. They give no guarantees—only positive facts about my particular cancer. I keep looking for evidence that hope is reasonable. Little by little it's becoming easier for me to be hopeful.

"One of my disadvantages is that I know too much. I know my disease. I've had patients who have done very well. But I've also had patients who have died, in spite of treatment. It's a comfort to realize how fast treatment today is improving.

"Still, that battle between hope and doubt rages within me. One day I'm full of hope, and the next I'm not too sure. I need the reassurance that comes from my medical team. I'm learning that a doctor's judgment in his own case is worth very little. I do know, though, that I'm safe right now. I don't know what the future holds."

> O LORD, how many are my foes!
>   How many rise up against me!
> Many are saying of me,
>   "God will not deliver him."
>
> But you are a shield around me, O LORD;
>   you bestow glory on me and lift up my head.
> To the LORD I cry aloud,
>   and he answers me from his holy hill.
>
> I lie down and sleep;
>   I wake again, because the LORD sustains me.
> I will not fear the tens of thousands
>   drawn up against me on every side.
>
> Arise, O LORD!
>   Deliver me, O my God!
> Strike all my enemies on the jaw;
>   break the teeth of the wicked.
>
> From the LORD comes deliverance.
>   May your blessing be on your people.
>
> —David
> Psalm 3

In his book *The Cancer Conqueror* (Word, 1990), Greg Anderson lists ten positive beliefs about cancer, cancer treatment, and the patient's role. These beliefs are worth reading, meditating on, and worth making your own.

1. I do not believe cancer is synonymous with death.
2. I believe cancer cells are weak and confused; they don't eat other cells.
3. I believe treatment is very effective against these weak and confused cells.
4. I believe the side effects, if any, can be controlled.
5. I believe my own immune system overcomes cancer cells daily.
6. I believe I am personally responsible for my cancer journey.
7. I believe I manage my total treatment program.
8. I believe I am "cancering." It is a process I can master.
9. I believe I can control the emotional, psychological, and spiritual aspects of the illness.
10. I believe cancer is a message for me to change.

Why, who makes much of a miracle?
As to me I know of nothing else but miracles,
Whether I walk the streets of Manhattan,
Or dart my sight over the roofs of houses toward the sky,
Or wade with naked feet along the beach just in the edge
    of the water,
Or stand under trees in the woods,
Or talk by day with any one I love, or sleep in the bed at
    night with anyone I love,
Or sit at table at dinner with the rest,
Or look at strangers opposite me riding in the car,
Or watch honeybees busy around the hive of a summer
    forenoon,

Or animals feeding in the fields,
Or birds, or the wonderfulness of insects in the air,
Or the wonderfulness of the sundown, or of stars shining
    so quiet and bright,
Or the exquisite delicate thin curve of the new moon in
    spring;
These with the rest, one and all, are to me miracles,
The whole referring, yet each distinct and in its place.

To me every hour of the night and dark is a miracle,
Every cubic inch of space is a miracle,
Every square yard of the surface of the earth is spread with
    the same,
Every foot of the interior swarms with the same.

To me the sea is a continual miracle,
The fishes that swim—the rocks—the motion of the
    waves—the ships with men in them,
What stranger miracles are there?

      —Walt Whitman
      "Miracles"

"Patience" is a word that sounds pale, almost sickly. It suggests a wilted person; an empty person, crushed by life, marking time because it's no use struggling any more. Patience is such a passive grace.

In English, perhaps. But in the language of the Bible? Never! In Scripture "patience" has a bold, courageous ring. To communicate it requires several Hebrew and Greek words, but the underlying meaning of "patience" is "confident endurance." The patient man is undefeated. He stands firm, buffeted by life, but quietly persistent in doing good.

We need to understand what patience means. When our

197

toddlers annoy, patience reminds us that we can endure, and remain calm. When our efforts fail, patience reminds us that we need not surrender, but can still overcome. When others misunderstand or accuse us, patience reminds us that grace is longsuffering, and so we can keep on caring. When illness tempts us to despair and doubt, patience reminds us that healing is a process that often requires liberal use of time.

—Larry Richards
The Believer's Guidebook

The brave man is not he who feels no fear,
For that were stupid and irrational;
But he whose noble soul its fear subdues,
And bravely dares the danger nature shrinks from.

—Joanna Baillie
Eighteenth-century poet

O Love Divine, that stooped to share
    Our sharpest pang, our bitterest tear,
On Thee we cast each earth-born care,
    We smile at pain while Thou art near!

Though long the weary way we tread,
    And sorrow crown each lingering year,
No path we shun, no darkness dread,
    Our hearts still whispering, Thou art near!

When drooping pleasure turns to grief,
    And trembling faith is changed to fear,

198

UNCERTAINTY

The murmuring wind, the quivering leaf,
  Shall softly tell us, Thou art near!

On Thee we fling our burdening woe,
  O Love Divine, forever dear,
Content to suffer while we know,
  Living and Dying, Thou art near!
                    —Oliver Wendell Holmes
                    "Hymn of Trust"

Cultivating a positive attitude is key to a sensible anticancer strategy. Whether through visualization techniques (in which you imagine your immune system overpowering the disease) or the support of loving friends or family members, anything that lifts your spirits and gives you hope is a positive move.

An unmeasurable, unquantifiable, vital aspect of fighting cancer is what I call Factor X. It's hope, or a sense of control over fate, or a feeling of actively taking part in the skirmishes against cancer. These are the things that can enhance our sense of well-being, our ability to cope with the ordeal of disease, our willingness to comply with the rigors of medical treatment.
                    —Robert Rodale
                    Prevention Magazine, May 1989

Prayer
Lord, help me starve my doubts and exercise my hope.

RESIGNATION

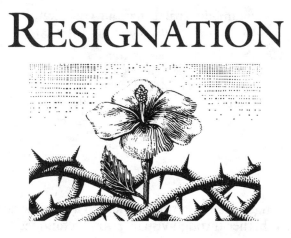

"I find I'm resigned to the fact that I am a cancer victim. I guess I may as well make the best of it. I've known about this disease for so long. But I haven't really *known* it until now. As a matter of fact, I've finally begun to realize that I'm fortunate. I mean, lymphoma is one of the better cancers as far as modern treatment is concerned. I should be thankful. But somehow I can't quite bring myself to that.

"I'm thankful for the state of the art in diagnosing and treating my tumor. I've also gotten to the place where I realize I'm no better than anyone else. As long as these things are around, it might as well be me as someone else.

"My thinking is getting clearer, and I can read the newspaper again. I do have flashbacks now and then, times when I feel confused and isolated. But at least when that happens, I realize now that I'm 'out of order.' I know it will be temporary.

"I'm not mad about this happening. And I'm not accusing God and asking 'Why did you do this to *me?*' I guess I'm even resigned to the fact that my private life has been invaded and my routine interrupted. I can't get up and go in to work, so I guess I may as well buckle down and get on with battling my cancer."

Kenneth Patchen, a contemporary poet who became bedridden with a painful and disabling spinal disease in 1960, understands the struggle between doubt and hope, anger and praise. He shares that struggle in a poem he calls

THE EVERLASTING CONTENDERS

Of the beast . . . an angel
Creatures of the earth
It is good
Any who praise not grandly

O but they should

But they should
Death waits for everything that lives
Beast of the wood
Grim beast of the wood

Who praise not grandly

Should should
Heart weeps for all things
Here
And is greatly comforted
For heart is the angel
Of all
Who praise not grandly

But wish they could

CONQUERING CANCER

Have the courage to live. Anyone can die.
—Robert Cody

Oh, yet we trust that somehow good
   Will be the final goal of ill,
   To pangs of nature, sins of will,
Defects of doubt, and taints of blood;

That nothing walks with aimless feet;
   That not one life shall be destroyed
   Or cast as rubbish to the void,
When God hath made the pile complete;

That not a worm is cloven in vain;
   That not a moth with vain desire
   Is shriveled in a fruitless fire,
Or but subserves another's gain.

Behold, we know not anything;
   I can but trust that good shall fall
   At last—far off—at last, to all,
And every winter change to spring.

—Alfred Lord Tennyson
from "In Memoriam"

Ask and it will be given to you; seek and you will find;
knock and the door will be opened to you. For everyone who

asks receives; he who seeks finds; and to him who knocks, the door will be opened.

Which of you, if his son asks for bread, will give him a stone? Or if he asks for a fish, will give him a snake? If you, then, though you are evil, know how to give good gifts to your children, how much more will your Father in heaven give good gifts to those who ask him!

—Jesus Christ
Matthew 7:7–11

When a man finds no peace within himself it is useless to seek it elsewhere.

—LaRochefoucauld

Out of suffering have emerged the strongest souls; the most massive characters are seared with scars.

—E. H. Chapin

Prayer

Lord, help me to make the best of my cancer. And, Lord, help my cancer to make your very best of me.

COURAGE

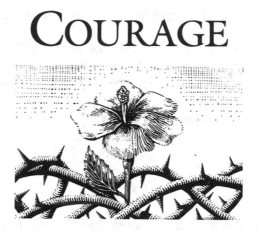

"As a doctor, I've advised many patients with life-threatening conditions to take life a day at a time. That is, to live in "day tight compartments." That certainly wasn't original with me. Jesus gave that wise advice centuries ago, when he said, "Do not worry about tomorrow, for tomorrow will worry about itself" (Matt. 6:34). To me, that means not wasting time fussing and stewing over things I can't do anything about. I need to do everything that's expected of me to further my cause, and then put it to rest.

"That's easier for some to do than for others. We all have our pet weaknesses. I'm pretty good at the 'if only's.' I've practiced for years! But there are no 'if only's' now.

"So I've become a pretty good patient. I trust my team of doctors. I do what they tell me. I keep them informed of how I'm feeling, and they keep a close check on my blood count. There are day-to-day zigs and zags in my treatment and in how I'm feeling. But I have to take it day by day. I guess that's a pretty good definition of courage: Taking life day by day, fighting each day's battle and not worrying about tomorrow."

Therefore I tell you, do not worry about your life, what you will eat or drink; or about your body, what you will wear. Is not life more important than food, and the body more important than clothes? Look at the birds of the air; they do not sow or reap or store away in barns, and yet your heavenly Father feeds them. Are you not much more valuable than they? Who of you by worrying can add a single hour to his life?

And why do you worry about clothes? See how the lilies of the field grow. They do not labor or spin. Yet I tell you that not even Solomon in all his splendor was dressed like one of these. If that is how God clothes the grass of the field, which is here today and tomorrow is thrown into the fire, will he not much more clothe you, O you of little faith? So do not worry, saying, "What shall we eat?" or "What shall we drink?" or "What shall we wear?" For the pagans run after all these things, and your heavenly Father knows that you need them. But seek first his kingdom and his righteousness, and all these things will be given to you as well. Therefore do not worry about tomorrow, for tomorrow will worry about itself. Each day has enough trouble of its own.

—Jesus Christ
Matthew 6:25–34

This time of learning new roles is often an uncomfortable one. When one member of a family is ill, relationships in a family often change. The financial provider may no longer work, the person responsible for cooking or driving children to school may be unable to do so, or a grandmother may "drop everything" to care for the children. A ripple effect can take place when a dependent person is catapulted into a role of responsibility, or when an independent head of a family relinquishes that role.

If you no longer can perform some or all of your former tasks, you may feel depressed and worthless. Many family members would rather not have to assume new responsibilities, some take it in their stride, and a few may become bossy in their new role.

Changes in roles can occur suddenly or develop gradually over a period of time. Family members who remain sensitive to underlying meanings may be able to minimize the emotional impact. For instance, people who can no longer shop or cook may still feel they maintain control over the kitchen if they can plan the meals, make out the marketing list, and provide recipes. Those who can no longer go to work and bring home a paycheck can still do much of the family budgeting and find useful tasks to do at home.

You and your family will cope best with these changes if you realize that *you* haven't changed but are just performing new and different jobs.

—Marion Morra and Eve Potts
Choices

Being a man, ne'er ask the gods for life set free from grief, but ask for courage that endureth long.

—Menander
Greek dramatist

COURAGE

Against the day of sorrow
Lay by some trifling thing
A smile, a kiss, a flower
For sweet remembering.

Then when the day is darkest
Without one rift of blue
Take out your little trifle
And dream your dream anew.

—Georgia Douglas Johnson
"Trifle"

Fear, we are told, should be overcome. But we face legitimate fears as well as unhealthy ones.

Unhealthy fears distort reality or are overreactions to possible dangers. For instance, the fear that I'll have some overwhelming pain in the future is an unhealthy fear. It keeps me anxious and upset, even though I don't feel pain now, and even though I'm assured if pain comes, my doctors have medication to control it.

Legitimate fears are closely linked with realities. Fire burns, and children must learn not to touch it. Cancer can kill, and so I muster every resource to combat it. How much better it is to face this fear than to deny or repress my uncertainties.

Several practices can help us deal with fears that are related to real threats, like cancer.

- Accept the reality of the threat and don't try to deny it.
- Accept your own feelings of fear as legitimate.

- Gather information that will help you deal with the threat realistically. Knowing what to expect can help avoid panic.
- Don't be afraid of fear, but use it to motivate you to take a daily step that will help you overcome the threat.

Be strong and courageous.
Do not be afraid or terrified
because of them,
for the LORD your God
goes with you;
he will never leave you
nor forsake you.

—Moses
Deuteronomy 31:6

It boils down to just one thing: Do I face the fact that I *choose* to do, and to be, what I am?

Blaming others or fate may seem to offer an easy way out. But the fact is that each of us bears personal responsibility for every act.

I can't choose today what I did yesterday. I can't even choose today what I will do tomorrow. But I can choose, this minute, what I will think and do now.

By what I choose now, I shape my tomorrows.

By what I choose today, I construct the yesterdays I will live with all my life.

By taking control in my today, by accepting the privilege

and responsibility of daily choice, I forge the past and future I will live with all my life.

Prayer

Lord, free me from the paralyzing effects of fear that I may walk boldly in this "today" and take the steps that will lead me to a brighter tomorrow.

Searching

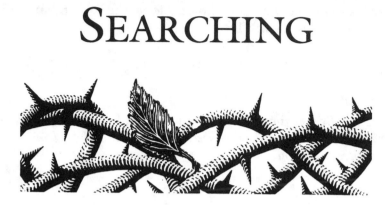

"Every cancer is different in some respect. So I've been reading everything I can find about lymphomas and the progress in managing them. Anyone can do this. If there's something they don't understand, they can ask their doctors. I've found that an educated patient is much easier to treat successfully than one who knows little about the issue.

"Now, my tumor has spread beyond the surgical field. They couldn't remove it all because the nodes around the aorta were involved. It was impossible to remove the entire tumor without injuring the aorta, so there is definitely some cancer left behind. I just have to do something else, or my days are numbered!

"My sister-in-law, a doctor in Bakersfield, knew one of the leaders in the treatment of lymphoma at Stanford University. My doctors cooperated and sent all my records up to him. He was very comfortable in discussing any aspect of my disease, and he had the answers.

"We've all got a right to search for answers. And to get them from our doctors. How I appreciate the willingness of everyone to help me as I'm searching for insights and answers into my care."

I didn't sleep much. I couldn't, somehow, for thinking. And every time I waked up I thought somebody had me by the neck. So the sleep didn't do me no good. By and by I says to myself, I can't live this way; I'm a-going to find out who it is that's here on the island with me; I'll find it out or bust. Well, I felt better right off.

—Huckleberry Finn
The Adventures of Huckleberry Finn
Mark Twain

The beginning of health is to know the disease.

—Cervantes
Don Quixote

"I came from an old-fashioned family where the father was the breadwinner and the mother stayed home and took care of the household. She became the center of things that went on at home. My brother and I were really lucky to have the stability and love that radiated from her. She made everything okay and gave us a security that seemed invincible. She could take care of anything, and my home was a real haven, where none of the bad stuff of the outside world could invade.

"It was a tremendous shock when I received a phone call at

college that my mother had been operated on for cancer of the ovary and it was impossible to remove it all. This was the first time in my life that I had been faced with a tragedy in my own family. It had always happened to the other guy before, but now it was my turn. How was I to handle this crisis? Not very well, I'm here to tell you. My perfect world had been threatened at the very core. Cancer and all of its ugliness had been brought to me personally. Nothing looked right at the time. The flowers didn't look too beautiful, the birds sang flat, food was dull. The whole world was uncomfortable. For the first time I was seeing the real world, and this part of it I didn't like.

"None of us likes it, but we are all in the same boat. Sickness and death are enemies, and we want to avoid them as long as possible. Of all the diseases I studied and lived with, cancer has been the most ominous and threatening. Nearly every family has been touched by cancer. If you deny that, you just don't know your family very well. Cancer is omnipresent. Fortunately, we are closing in on the cause and the prevention of this scourge."

You've got time: We've all heard that early *diagnosis* of cancer saves lives. An early-stage cancer—one that hasn't started to spread throughout the body—is easier to treat. But no cancer spreads so rapidly that you don't have some time to check your treatment options. In fact, you may jeopardize the success of your treatment if you don't take the time to think things through. "The initial treatment is the most important one," says John E. Ultmann, M.D., director of the University of Chicago Cancer Research Center. "It's your best chance for a successful outcome."

—Special Report
Prevention Magazine
May 1989

Consider it pure joy, my brothers, whenever you face trials of many kinds, because you know that the testing of your faith develops perseverance. Perseverance must finish its work so that you may be mature and complete, not lacking anything. If any of you lacks wisdom, he should ask God, who gives generously to all without finding fault, and it will be given to him. But when he asks, he must believe and not doubt, because he who doubts is like a wave of the sea, blown and tossed by the wind.

—James
James 1:2–6

The disciplined person is the person who can do what needs to be done when it needs to be done. The disciplined person is the person who can live in the appropriateness of the hour. The extreme ascetic and the glutton have exactly the same problem: they cannot do what needs to be done when it needs to be done. The disciplined person is the free person.

—Richard J. Foster
Reasons to Be Glad

Be strong and courageous. Do not be terrified; do not be discouraged, for the LORD your God will be with you wherever you go.

—God speaking to Joshua
Joshua 1:9

Prayer

Lord, remind me of my ABC's. Help me be assertive, bold, and constant in my search for answers.

COMFORT

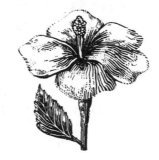

"I've been amazed, now that my diagnosis is certain and I'm into treatment, how many people are in the same boat. It's as if we have a special club, with members all having the same problem. We're all the same, and yet different, because each case is totally distinct.

"This is one reason cancer is so difficult to treat. What works for one person may not work for the other. Still, there are enough similarities so treatments can be standardized and the differences can be intelligently and adequately dealt with.

"Really, it's kind of a confidence builder to run into other people with a similar problem and know they're under a treatment that's working. It's surprising to discover how much you can learn from others. And it's comforting to feel that you're not alone."

TEN COMMANDMENTS FOR FRIENDS AND FAMILY

1. Don't give me medical advice.
2. Don't keep asking me how I feel or telling me how I *should* feel.
3. Don't tell me about other cancer patients who haven't made it.
4. Don't belittle my problem or give false reassurance.
5. Don't avoid me, but be available.
6. Listen to me when I want to talk, and ask me for advice about matters in which I'm knowledgeable. I have a lot to contribute even though I'm sick.
7. Sometimes just sit quietly with me. You don't have to talk constantly to be a comfort.
8. Don't let me feel abandoned, but realize that sometimes I just need to be alone.
9. Always be hopeful for me. I need your reassurance.
10. Provide spiritual support.

—Paul Johnson

I think it frets the saints in heaven to see
How many desolate creatures on the earth
Have learnt the simple dues of fellowship
And social comfort, in a hospital.

—Elizabeth Barrett Browning
Aurora Leigh

216

Technical books about communication talk about encoding and decoding messages. But this doesn't help much when we're frustrated because no matter how hard we try, we can't seem to get others to understand what we're trying to say. What does help?

We need to make sure that we share on five different levels, levels that make understanding possible.

● *First-level information is what you receive from your senses.* To clarify how you understand, you may need to say specifically what you saw or heard or how you feel.

● *Second-level information is telling how you interpret what you saw or heard or feel.* "I have a pain in my left side" is first-level information. "I think my cancer is spreading" or "I think the medication must be working" tells how you interpret that pain.

● *Third-level information is how you* feel *about your interpretation of what you see, heard, or felt.* You may feel deepening anxiety if you think the pain signals a growth of the cancer, or you may feel excited if you're convinced the medication is working.

● *Fourth-level information is an expression of intention.* This means telling the other person how we want him or her to understand what we've said. Seeing a frightened look on the face of a spouse may lead us to say, "It's okay. I just feel a little anxious because I'm not sure about the side effects of my new medicine. I don't want you to think the pain is unbearable, because it's not."

● *Fifth-level information is action information; it communicates what we expect or want the other person to do.* For instance, "I don't think it's anything serious, but why don't you call the doctor and let me talk to him." Or, "Would you get me the *Conquering Cancer* book and see if what I feel is a possible side effect of my new medicine?"

When one or more of these five levels of communication is blocked, people operate blindly. Neither person really understands what is happening inside the other. A person may refuse to express his or her feeling. Or a person may never spell out intentions or say what action he or she would like the other person to take. When we fail to share such information, relationships are uncertain and strained, and the chance for real intimacy is lessened.

We especially need the comfort of being close to others when we're in a lengthy battle with cancer. So let's give our loved ones information on all five levels. And remember these questions that will help us *get* the sharing we need from others:

What makes you think that?
How do you feel about that?
What is it that you want?
What can we do about it?

Praise be to the God and Father of our Lord Jesus Christ, the Father of compassion and the God of all comfort, who comforts us in all our troubles, so that we can comfort those in any trouble with the comfort we ourselves have received from God. For just as the sufferings of Christ flow over into our lives, so also through Christ our comfort overflows. If we are distressed, it is for your comfort and salvation; if we are comforted, it is for your comfort, which produces in you patient endurance of the same sufferings we suffer. And our hope for you is firm, because we know that just as you share in our sufferings, so also you share in our comfort.

—Paul
2 Corinthians 1:3–7

Never say "I don't *have* any friends." The real issue is, *"Am I a friend?"*

—John Westerhoff III

comfort (kum'fort) 1. to soothe in distress or sorrow; ease the misery or grief of; bring consolation or hope to. 2. to give a sense of ease to.

—*Webster's New World Dictionary*

Without belittling the courage with which men have died, we should not forget those acts of courage with which men have *lived*.

—John F. Kennedy

Prayer

Lord, I ask not to be comfortable, but to be comforted and to be a comforter.

GROWING CONFIDENCE

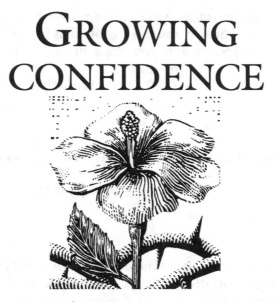

"At last I can feel my resignation being replaced by confidence. I now feel that I have a chance to get well. In fact, I don't even think about *not* getting well!

"I'm back to work again. Not that I'm superman. I don't stay at the office all day. And I don't do any surgery yet. I'm just not up to that. But I'm puttering around the office, and being around familiar things and people is a real boost to me.

"I've come a long way and am getting stronger every day. I'm now taking daily X-ray treatments and go to the hospital by myself. I'm getting back my confidence, and I feel that everyone is pulling for me. Order is emerging from my time of chaos.

"Not long ago I felt totally defeated and alone. Now things are changing. I can smile again and face the future with confidence, even though the outcome cannot be guaranteed."

Remember this also, and be well persuaded of its truth; the future is not in hands of Fate, but in ours.

—Jules Jusserand

Marcie McS., age six, is just about to undergo a bone-marrow transplant to cure her leukemia. Ten years ago such transplants weren't even possible, and Marcie would surely have died. Just two years ago, the chances that a bone-marrow transplant would "take" were only about fifty-fifty—a terrible risk to face. But today, due to a new, experimental method of treating bone-marrow transplant cells, the odds in Marcie's favor are greatly increased, and her doctors now believe she has an excellent chance of winning her fight against cancer.

Carol T., age fifty-three, was diagnosed with lung cancer three years ago. Even after successful surgery, her chances of long-term survival without recurrence were only about ten percent. But thanks to a sophisticated new form of post-operative immunotherapy recently developed, Carol has already survived three times as long as most patients in her situation, with no sign of recurrence.

Although it sometimes seems as if progress against this disease is discouragingly slow, in truth, scientists are reporting promising results at an exciting pace.

—*Good Housekeeping*
November 1988

Physicians consider that when the cause of a disease is discovered, the cure is discovered.

—Cicero

Some cancer patients remind me of the peddler from the legendary European Jewish town of Khelm, inhabited by endearing but none-too-wise people. This peddler, carrying a heavy pack, was picked up by a farmer who was riding home in his wagon. The peddler sat down by the farmer but kept the pack on his shoulder.

When asked why he didn't take the pack off his shoulder and give himself a rest, the peddler shrugged. "It's nice enough that your horse is *schlepping* me. Why should I add my bundle to his burden?"

Saying "thank you" may seem like a strange way to gain relief from the burden of anxiety. But it really helps. Take a few minutes each day and write a note to just one of the many people on the medical team that is treating your cancer. It may be a note to one of your doctors, an X-ray technician, an office nurse. Perhaps it's a word of appreciation for his or her skill. Perhaps thanks for a smile, a friendly word, a caring look or touch. Taking time to write will do more than make you and the recipient feel positive and warm. It will remind you of the team that is working with you to win a victory over your

222

cancer. Unlike the peddler in the old Yiddish story, you'll realize more clearly with each note that you really can relax a bit and set your burden down.

> Two roads diverged in a yellow wood,
> And sorry I could not travel both
> And be one traveler, long I stood
> And looked down one as far as I could
> To where it bent in the undergrowth;
>
> Then took the other, as just as fair,
> And having perhaps the better claim,
> Because it was grassy and wanted wear;
> Though as for that the passing there
> Had worn them really about the same,
>
> And both that morning equally lay
> In leaves no step had trodden black.
> Oh, I kept the first for another day!
> Yet knowing how way leads on to way,
> I doubted if I should ever come back.
>
> I shall be telling this with a sigh
> Somewhere ages and ages hence:
> Two roads diverged in a wood, and I—
> I took the one less traveled by,
> And that has made all the difference.
>
> —Robert Frost
> "The Road Not Taken"

CONQUERING CANCER

Cast all your anxiety on him because he cares for you.
—Peter
1 Peter 5:7

Prayer

Thank you for the gift of those who, like you, care for me as I walk this road.

STRETCHING

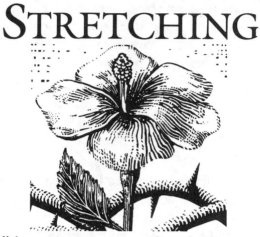

"I'm well into my treatment and am having some ups and downs. That chemotherapy makes me feel lousy with nausea. I vomit, my hair is falling out, and my hands and fingers are a little numb.

"Sometimes I wonder if it's really worth it. Is this all there is? Peggy Lee's song becomes more real by the day. This is an adventure I hadn't bargained for.

"The medicine my doctor gives me helps a little. I have to work to remember that I'm not alone, that anything worthwhile is worth struggling for.

"Sure, I'm paying a price. But it won't be long until I can look back on the whole thing. Even now my tests show that what's left of my tumor is just half the size it was when we started.

"Is it worth it? You know it is!"

We also rejoice in our sufferings, because we know that

suffering produces perseverance; perseverance, character; and character, hope. And hope does not disappoint us, because God has poured out his love into our hearts by the Holy Spirit, whom he has given to us.

—Paul
Romans 5:3–5

Sometimes it's helpful to have a Pity Party. You just decide you're going to spend some time getting it all out of your system. Decide you'll spend a full hour thinking about how bad things are and focusing on your sufferings. Here are some helpful hints.

The best time to schedule a Pity Party is when you'd rather be doing something else—watching TV, eating a snack, reading, even sleeping. It's also important to make sure the place you choose for your Pity Party is as sterile as possible. Maybe a straight chair, in an airless, dark room. You'll also want to select an uncomfortable position. Try standing in a corner, or sit cross-legged on the floor—maybe even in a closet. And if you can, see the place is too hot or too cold to be enjoyable.

I know. This sounds silly. Still, there's no sense *enjoying* self-pity. So be creative in making your Pity Party as unrewarding as possible. After a few days of serious effort you may decide that you don't enjoy indulging in self-pity after all. You may even find yourself looking ahead, thinking about all those positive things you can do to make your present situation more pleasant. And your future more secure.

STRETCHING

I have been one acquainted with the night.
I have walked out in rain—and back in rain.
I have outwalked the furthest city light.

I have looked down the saddest city lane.
I have passed by the watchman on his beat
And dropped my eyes, unwilling to explain.

I have stood still and stopped the sound of feet
When far away an interrupted cry
Came over houses from another street,

But not to call me back to say good-by;
And further still at an unearthly height,
One luminary clock against the sky

Proclaimed the time was neither wrong nor right,
I have been one acquainted with the night.

> —Robert Frost
> "Acquainted with the Night"

To be willing to suffer in order to create is one thing; to realize that one's creation necessitates one's suffering, that suffering is one of the greatest of God's gifts, is almost to reach a mystical solution of the problem of evil.

> —J.W.N. Sullivan

CONQUERING CANCER

My wounds fester and are loathsome
  because of my sinful folly.
I am bowed down and brought very low;
  all day long I go about mourning.
My back is filled with searing pain;
  there is no health in my body.
I am feeble and utterly crushed;
  I groan in anguish of heart.

All my longings lie open before you, O Lord;
  my sighing is not hidden from you.
My heart pounds, my strength fails me;
  even the light has gone from my eyes.
My friends and companions avoid me because of my
    wounds;
  my neighbors stay far away.

I am like a deaf man, who cannot hear,
  like a mute, who cannot open his mouth;
I have become like a man who does not hear,
  whose mouth can offer no reply.
I wait for you, O Lord;
  you will answer, O Lord my God.
For I said, "Do not let them gloat
  or exalt themselves over me when my foot slips."

O Lord, do not forsake me;
  be not far from me, O my God.
Come quickly to help me,
  O Lord my Savior.

                —David
                from Psalm 38

STRETCHING

If you suffer, thank God!—it is a sure sign that you are alive.

—Elbert Hubbard

I want to be heard.
    Hear me, as I hear you,
    Listen, I'm listening to you.

So I will speak simply
    with clear word windows
    that let you see
    all the way in
    to where I live
        laugh
        and
        cry.

—David Augsburger
Caring Enough to Confront

Prayer
God grant me the serenity
To accept things I cannot change,
Courage to change things I can,
And the wisdom to know the difference.

—Reinhold Niebuhr

SETTING GOALS

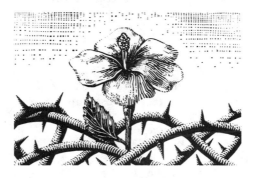

"From the first time I set foot in the hospital, I began having goals.

"The first one was to get out of the hospital.

"That came and went.

"The next was to get outside, walking. And that happened.

"I remember the big one. Getting back to the office. Just getting into the office was such a morale booster, even though I didn't do anything.

"My resistance to cancer is building, and with each goal I attain, the memory of the bad things about my disease is being erased. It's amazing how soon we forget the miserable things about our course of treatment when a few goals are attained."

Everyone agrees we need to set goals. "Shoot at nothin'," the old farmer is supposed to have said, "an' you'll be sure to hit it." I know I need to set goals. If I didn't, I suspect I would get a lot less done. But only some approaches to setting goals are productive. Here are some guidelines.

● Set goals for level of activity, not for results. I can put in a disciplined effort, but I can't guarantee results. Actually, setting result goals may create unnecessary guilt. When I set goals for myself, I am disciplining myself to faithfulness. I need to be faithful. Let God worry about the results.

● Set goals as guidelines, not masters. If you aren't able to reach the goals you set or if something unexpected intrudes, don't get upset. Revise your goals.

● Set goals for now, not for years to come. Goals are helpful in developing discipline for present tasks. Reaching a short-term goal, even if it's something so simple as getting dressed and sitting up for half an hour, is a measure of progress and a real encouragement. When we reach a goal like getting back to work or preparing a meal for the family, we *know* we're getting better.

To sum it up, set goals that bring personal discipline to your present activities and that lead you step by step in the good future that lies ahead.

As a cure for worrying, work is better than whiskey.

—Thomas A. Edison

Brothers, I do not consider myself yet to have taken hold of it. But one thing I do: Forgetting what is behind and straining toward what is ahead, I press on toward the goal to win the prize for which God has called me heavenward in

Christ Jesus. All of us who are mature should take such a view of things.

—Paul
Philippians 3:13–15a

Those who plan what is good find love and faithfulness.
—Solomon
Proverbs 14:22

Work is a grand cure for all the maladies and miseries that ever beset mankind—honest work, which you intend getting done.

—Thomas Carlyle

One of the old prophets wrote, "Do not despise the day of small things." He was talking about that very human trait of looking around, seeing how little progress we're making, and then getting so discouraged we quit.

Conquering cancer is filled with days of small things. Taking that extra bite of food when our appetite is gone. Going those few extra steps when we're suddenly totally exhausted. Making the effort to prepare a salad for the family, when that's all we can manage of our old role as chief cook and bottle washer.

It's a tragic mistake if we compare what we can do now, while recovering from our treatments, with what we could do before. When we do, our present capacities seem so small, so insignificant. But what the prophet realized, and what we need to understand, is that the day of small things isn't to be despised. Each day of small steps toward regaining our strength, each day of just a little more progress toward even limited goals moves us in the direction we simply have to go: the direction of recovery. The day of big things—health and wholeness—lies ahead!

A goal you can achieve is better than a dream that is beyond reach.

Prayer
Lord, help me sense the importance of the step I take today. Keep me from discouragement about how far I have yet to go.

SENSITIVITY

"I love to watch the family of wood ducks cruising by our dock. They've been here for years. But somehow the bold pattern of their feathers seems sharper and clearer these days. I watch the sun dance on the waters of Lake Washington, as Mount Rainier floats like a mirage in the distance. The mountain seems to float peacefully in the sky, only its snowy peak and rugged shoulders visible.

"I've always enjoyed nature. But now that I've been keeping company with death, the world around me seems more vibrantly alive.

"As I am.

"It's so easy to take God's gifts for granted. Coming out the other side of what Psalm 23 calls the 'valley of the shadow of death,' I've discovered a new sensitivity to what is most important in life. A loving touch. The caress of a passing breeze. Rain dancing on the deck outside my window. A wood duck, paddling by in grand preoccupation."

SENSITIVITY

A personal discovery I am just coming into is the joy and touch of real living that comes with "celebrating the temporary." Stopping to notice and drink more deeply of *now*.

The past is past. I can learn from it but I cannot relive it. The future is to be prepared for, but I cannot live there either. Today—this moment—I have.

Now is not just a tiny, pinched, confining crevice between yesterday and tomorrow. Now is life. The only bit of life I have.

Lord, I want to live open and full and awake *now*. Remind me to smell the roses in front of my house . . . now, today. Remind me to hug my kids and my wife and tell them I love them . . . today. Remind me to breathe—I mean *really* breathe . . . today.

> —Bob Girard
> *My Weakness: His Strength*

Whither, midst falling dew,
While glow the heavens with the last steps of day,
Far, through their rosy depths, dost thou persue
    Thy solitary way?

Vainly the fowler's eye
Might mark thy distant flight to do thee wrong,
As, darkly seen against the crimson sky,
    Thy figure floats along.

Seek'st thou the plashy brink
Of weedy lake, or marge of river wide,

235

Or where the rocking billows rise and sink
  On the chafed oceanside?

There is a Power whose care
Teaches thy way along the pathless coast—
The desert and illimitable air—
  Lone wandering, but not lost.

All day thy wings have fanned,
At that far height, the cold, thin atmosphere,
Yet stoop not, weary, to the welcome land,
  Though the dark night is near.

And soon that toil shall end;
Soon shalt thou find a summer home, and rest,
And scream among thy fellows; reeds shall bend,
  Soon, o'er thy sheltered nest.

Thou'rt gone, the abyss of heaven
Hath swallowed up thy form; yet, on my heart
Deeply hath sunk the lesson thou hast given,
  And shall not soon depart.

He who, from zone to zone,
Guides through the boundless sky thy certain flight,
In the long way that I must tread alone,
  Will lead my steps aright.

> —William Cullen Bryant
> "To a Waterfowl"

There is a pleasure in the pathless woods,
There is a rapture on the lonely shore,
There is society, where none intrudes,
By the deep sea and music in its roar:
I love not man the less, but Nature more,

236

SENSITIVITY

From these our interviews, in which I steal
From all I may be, or have been before,
To mingle with the Universe, and feel
What I can ne'er express, yet cannot all conceal.

—Lord Byron
"Sonnet 178"

I could not walk this darkening path of pain alone.
The years have taken toll of me;
Sometimes my banners droop, my arms have grown
too tired,
And laughter comes less easily.

And often these my shrinking cowardly eyes refuse
To face the thing that is ahead of me,
The certainty of growing pain and helplessness . . .
But O, my Lord is good, for He

Comes quickly to me as I lie there in the dust
Of my defeat and shame and fear.
He stoops and raises me, and sets me on my feet,
And softly whispers in my ear

That He will never leave me—nay, that He will go
Before me all the way. And so,
My hand in His, along this brightening path of pain,
My Lord and I together go.

—Martha Snell Nicholson
"When He Putteth Forth His
Own Sheep, He Goeth Before
Them"

237

CONQUERING CANCER

I know it sounds corny, but somehow the sun seems brighter and the grass seems greener these days. I always loved to walk in the park near our house, but often I was too busy to find time. Now I still have the same job and home obligations, but I find time to walk in the park almost every day. I know they haven't done any landscaping there recently, but every tree and little bush looks more beautiful than ever. I enjoy watching the seasons change, treasuring each one, but also looking forward to the next.

Lest you think I'm some kind of saint, you should know that I have terrible crying jags at times, get into loud arguments with my husband, and drive the kids crazy about keeping their rooms neat.

Still, a postcard or a phone call from a friend I haven't seen for a while seems very precious. I guess you might say life suddenly seems sweeter now that I know it's no longer guaranteed.

—A cancer patient

As a fond mother, when the day is o'er,
  Leads by the hand her little child to bed,
  Half willing, half reluctant to be led,
  And leave his broken playthings on the floor,
Still gazing at them through the open door,
  Nor wholly reassured and comforted
  By promises of others in their stead,
  Which, though more splendid, may not please him more;
So Nature deals with us, and takes away

238

SENSITIVITY

Our playthings one by one, and by the hand
Leads us to rest so gently, that we go
Scarce knowing if we wish to go or stay,
Being too full of sleep to understand
How far the unknown transcends what we know.

Author unknown

Praise the LORD, O my soul.

O LORD my God, you are very great;
    you are clothed with splendor and majesty.
He wraps himself in light as with a garment;
    he stretches out the heavens like a tent
    and lays the beams of his upper
        chambers in their waters.

He makes the clouds his chariot
    and rides on the wings of the wind.
He makes winds his messengers,
    flames of fire his servants.

He make springs pour water into the ravines;
    it flows between the mountains.
They give water to all the beasts of the field;
    the wild donkeys quench their thirst.
The birds of the air nest by the waters,
    they sing among the branches.
He waters the mountains from his upper chambers;
    the earth is satisfied by the fruit of his work.
He makes grass grow for the cattle,
    and plants for man to cultivate—
    bringing forth food from the earth:
wine that gladdens the heart of man,

oil to make his face shine,
and bread that sustains his heart.

How many are your works, O LORD!
In wisdom you made them all;
the earth is full of your creatures.
—from Psalm 104

Prayer

O God, calm my troubled heart with the beauty you have spread so liberally all around me.

THANKFULNESS

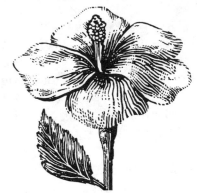

"I have so much to be thankful for.

"Death came calling and settled down in an easy chair next to me. Death waited, an unwelcome visitor, finding all sorts of excuses not to leave.

"How thankful I am for Genevieve, who held my hand. For my doctors, who supervised my treatment. For medicine itself, for the researchers and scientists who made the discoveries that made my successful treatment possible.

"How thankful I am for recovering myself. For my work, a work that offers me the privilege of serving others. How thankful I am for people, and for liking people.

"I'm not afraid to die. I believe eternal life is waiting for me when I close my eyes a final time. But, for now, how thankful I am that death finally gave up, got up out of my easy chair, and went out, slamming the door behind it in disappointment. Death will come visiting again, but only when it's time. Until then I'll appreciate the gift of added years that I've been given. And I'll be thankful."

There is nothing so effective in making the soul, body, and spirit function in a healthy and productive manner as being thankful. All of the healthy enzymes and hormones spring into action, and the whole *you* surges into a rightful position of dominion. For God created us to have dominion. So many times we forget, and even minimize, the blessings that we have. It's so easy just to take things for granted. With modern methods of communication, and bombardment by the media with bad news so many hours of the day, we seem to be immersed in pessimism and despair. It's very difficult to be thankful in this environment unless we consciously make an effort to extricate ourselves from the influence of the news media.

Being thankful in the morning just gets you off on the right foot. The smell of breakfast, a good appetite, a good night's sleep, freedom from pain, so many things we don't even think of. And then, the sun shining on the fresh leaves after a spring rain shower—the freshness of the air and the songs of the birds who are confirming your blessings. Consciously recognizing these little things is better than the best tonic in the world, and your systems respond by making you feel better all over. The mind is able to relax, and you begin to feel secure and confident.

That's how you were meant to feel. With wholeness, you can confront the abrasiveness of the world system. Thankfulness leads to joy, which leads to contentment, which certainly leads to fulfillment and satisfaction.

Life should be like that. And it can be.

THANKFULNESS

It is good to praise the LORD
   and make music to your name, O Most High,
to proclaim your love in the morning
   and your faithfulness at night,
to the music of the ten-stringed lyre
   and the melody of the harp.

For you make me glad by your deeds, O LORD;
   I sing for joy at the works of your hands.
How great are your works, O LORD,
   how profound your thoughts!

           —Psalm 92:1–5

Had you given in to me, Lord
On the thing I wanted so much,
My life today
Would be a sorry mess.
I tell you nothing new—
I simply repeat
What you told me
Long, long ago.
Finally today I see it—
From your point of view.
Thank you for not giving in to me,
Thank you most of all
For patiently waiting
For me to give in to you.

        —Ruth Harms Calkin
          "Thank You for Waiting"

But now, this is what the LORD says—
   he who created you, O Jacob,
   he who formed you, O Israel:
"Fear not, for I have redeemed you;
   I have summoned you by name; you are mine.
When you pass through the waters,
   I will be with you;
and when you pass through the rivers,
   they will not sweep over you.
When you walk through the fire,
   you will not be burned;
   the flames will not set you ablaze.
For I am the LORD, your God,
   the Holy One of Israel, your Savior."

                —Isaiah 43:1–3

An old man showed up at the back door of the house we were renting. Opening the door a few cautious inches, we saw his eyes were glassy and his furrowed face glistened with silver stubble. He clutched a wicker basket holding a few unappealing vegetables. He bid us good morning and offered his produce for sale. We were uneasy enough that we made a quick purchase to alleviate both our pity and our fear.

He returned the next week, introduced himself as Mr. Roth, the man who lived in the shack down the road. As our fears subsided, we got close enough to realize it wasn't alcohol but cataracts that marbleized his eyes. On subsequent visits, he would shuffle in, wearing two mismatched right shoes, and pull out a harmonica.

One visit he exclaimed, "The Lord is so good. I came out of my shack this morning and found a bag full of shoes and clothing on my porch."

"That's wonderful, Mr. Roth!" we said. "We're happy for you."

"You know what's even more wonderful?" he asked. "Just yesterday I met some people that could use them."

—Mark Todd
Leadership Magazine

Praise be to you, O LORD,
    God of our father Israel,
    from everlasting to everlasting.
Yours, O LORD, is the greatness and the power
    and the glory and the majesty and the splendor,
    for everything in heaven and earth is yours.
Yours, O LORD, is the kingdom;
    you are exalted as head over all.
Wealth and honor come from you;
    you are the ruler of all things.
In your hands are strength and power
    to exalt and give strength to all.
Now, our God, we give you thanks,
    and praise your glorious name.

—King David
1 Chronicles 29:10–13

You have made known to me the path of life;
you will fill me with joy in your presence,
with eternal pleasures at your right hand.
—David
Psalm 16:11

Prayer

Lord, help me to recognize your good gifts and be thankful.

WHERE TO FIND HELP

American Cancer Society

 The American Cancer Society offers education, research, and patient services. The address of the national headquarters is: American Cancer Society, 777 Third Avenue, New York, NY 10017. State and local units can be found in local telephone directories.

Cancer Information Service

 The Cancer Information Service is a national telephone inquiry system sponsored by the National Cancer Institute. Trained staff members provide data on causes of cancer, how to prevent cancer, new cancer treatments, availability of medical facilities, and the nearest Comprehensive Cancer Center. Their toll-free number is 1-800-4-CANCER.

Community Organizations

 Many communities via civic organizations and churches offer assistance to patients and their families. Local hospitals, churches, and cancer societies will have listings of these services.

Comprehensive Cancer Center Network

 The National Cancer Institute has designated comprehensive cancer centers throughout the United States.

The cancer centers carry out medical research as well as provide patient care and treatment. Investigational drugs, treatments, and diagnostic methods are often started here.

Leukemia Society of America
Local chapters throughout the United States provide information and financial assistance to people with leukemia, Hodgkin's Disease, or lymphoma. The address of the national headquarters is: 211 East 43rd Street, New York, NY 10017.

National Hospice Organization
This is a nonprofit, private organization dedicated to promoting and maintaining care for the terminally ill. Literature, films, and a directory of hospice programs are available through the organization by writing: 1901 North Fort Meyer Drive, Arlington, VA 22209.

Support and Self-Help
After—Ask A Friend About Reconstruction, 99 Park Avenue, New York, NY 10016. A volunteer group that provides support for women considering breast reconstruction.

Candlelighters Foundation, Suite 1011, 2025 I Street NW, Washington, D.C. 20006. An international organization that assists the parents of children who have cancer.

Encore is a YWCA sponsored group for breast cancer patients.

I Can Cope is an American Cancer Society sponsored educational program that provides psychological support and information to patients.

International Association of Laryngectomies is a rehab program for people who have had laryngectomies.

Reach to Recovery is a rehab program for women who have had mastectomies.

United Ostomy Association, Inc., 2001 West Beverly Boulevard, Los Angeles, CA 90057, provides information and support for people with ostomies.

GLOSSARY OF MEDICAL TERMS

Adenocarcinoma. A cancer originating in glandular tissue.

Amino acid. The building block of protein and the essential part of DNA, the proper arrangement of which gives it viability.

Anaplastic. Growing without structure; an anaplastic cell is one that reverts to an embryonic form.

Anesthesiologist. A doctor who specializes in anesthesia.

Antibiotics. Chemicals used against infection.

Apogene. The gene that controls cholesterol metabolism.

Autonomic processes. Physiologic activities that occur automatically, such as dilation of the pupils, secretion of digestive enzymes, etc.

B cell. A key player in the immune system; a white-blood cell that produces antibodies.

Beta rays. A type of X ray.

Biopsy. The removal and examination of tissue from the living body in order to establish a precise diagnosis.

Blood gases. Chiefly oxygen and carbon dioxide, which maintain tissue metabolism and acid-base balance.

Cancer antibodies. Specific antibodies produced to attack specific cancers. These will be developed through vaccines and possibly used for cancer treatment in the near future.

Carcinogenesis. Any agent that produces or incites cancer.

Catheter. A tubular, flexible, surgical instrument for withdrawing fluids from (or introducing fluids into) a cavity of the body. It is often placed into the bladder through the urethra to drain urine.

Chemotherapy. Cancer treatment that uses chemicals and hormones to deter the growth of cancerous cells.

Chromosome. A structure within the nucleus of each cell; each human cell contains 46 chromosomes, each of which carries genes that determine a person's hereditary characteristics.

Circulating nurse. The name given to the operating-room nurse who verifies the instrument and sponge count and who keeps the team supplied.

Clone. In microbiology, the asexual reproduction of a single cell.

Cobalt bomb. Used in therapy as a source of X ray.

Colon. The large bowel.

Colostomy. The surgical creation of an artificial anus.

Contamination. Soiling by contact with organisms, viruses, or radioactive material.

CT or CAT scan (Computerized Axial Tomography). A highly specialized series of X rays of internal body parts, recorded on a magnetic disk and processed by a mini-computer for reconstruction display.

Cystoscope. An instrument inserted into the bladder to aid visibility of and surgery on the bladder.

Depression of the bone marrow. A toxic effect of chemotherapy in which the blood-forming elements of the marrow no longer perform their normal function of making blood cells.

DNA (deoxyribonucleic acid). This acid, found at the center of every living cell, is considered to be the auto-reproducing component of chromosomes and many viruses. DNA is the storage place of hereditary characteristics.

Electrolytes. Substances that break down into ions in the blood, such as sodium chloride and potassium chloride.

En bloc. In a lump, as a whole.

Endorphins. A group of brain substances that bind to the opiate receptors of the brain and raise the pain threshold.

Epidermis. The outermost and nonvascular layer of the skin.

Fluoroscopy. Examination of tissues and deep structures of the body by X ray, using the fluoroscope, an apparatus that makes visible the shadows of X rays, which are projected on a fluorescent screen.

Gamma rays. A type of X ray.

Gene. The self-reproducing biologic unit of heredity located at a definite position on a particular chromosome.

Gene splicing. Removing a segment of a chromosome or gene and splicing in a segment from another.

Genetic code. The hereditary information contained in a set of chromosomes and genes.

Genetic engineering. The field of manipulating the genes and chromosomes to produce more and better antibodies, antitoxins, hormones, etc. The long-range goal is to develop the ability to eliminate defective genes.

Genetic fingerprinting. Every person has his or her own individual DNA that can be identified by examining any cell from blood, hair, skin, etc.

Genome (gene + chromosome). A complete set of hereditary factors contained in the chromosomes and genes of a mature sperm or ovum.

Granulocyte. A white blood cell that contains granules in the cytoplasm (the part of a cell that is not the nucleus).

253

Gynecologist. A doctor who treats diseases of the female genital tract.

Hormone. A chemical substance produced in the body by an organ or cells of an organ; hormones regulate a specific activity of a certain organ.

Imaging. A diagnostic process that outlines hidden tissue.

Immune system. A complex defense system consisting of highly specialized cells, including white blood cells, especially lymphocytes.

Incision. A cut made with a sharp instrument.

Interferon. A chemical produced by T cells (white blood cells). Interferon actively fights against certain infections and leukemias.

Interleukin. A chemical used to stimulate parts of the body's immune system. Interleukin is used to treat melanomas and certain other cancers.

Intravenous. Administering fluids or medication into a vein.

Kaposi's sarcoma. Malignant lesions involving the blood vessels and usually appearing on the toes or legs as purple or dark-brown plaques or nodules.

Kidneys. Located on each side of the spine, these bean-shaped organs filter urine and regulate the acid-base balance of the body.

Liver. This large organ located in the upper abdomen is known as the laboratory of the body; the liver secretes bile and plays a key role in the body's metabolism of carbohydrates and proteins.

Local recurrence. Reappearance of a cancer at the local site.

Lymph node. A small mass of tissue in the form of a swelling, knot, or protuberance, either normal or pathological, consisting of lymphocytes (white blood cells).

Lymphatics. Designating the lymphatic system.

Lymphocyte. White blood cells that are the principle cells of the immune system. Lymphocytes play many roles and can change from one to the other as the situation dictates.

Lymphokine and cytokines. Chemicals produced by T cells and used by the body to resist cancers, viruses, and bacteria.

Lymphoma. A tumor consisting of lymphocytes.

Macrophage-phagocyte. A large, mean-looking cell that acts like a scavenger by cleaning up debris left in the battle between bacteria or cancer cells and the immune cells.

Malignant. Tending to become progressively worse and to result in death. Having the properties of cancer.

Meiosis. The special form of cell division that results in the chromosome number reduced by half. Thus, meiosis provides a constancy of chromosome number from generation to generation by producing germ cells with 23 chromosomes.

Mesentery. A membranous fold attaching various organs to the body wall, such as the peritoneum, which attaches the bowel to the abdominal cavity.

Metastasis. The transfer of cancer from one organ or part to another not directly connected with it.

Metastatic recurrence. Reappearance of the cancer at a distant site.

Microbiologist. A research expert in DNA, molecular biology, and genetic engineering.

Monoclonal. Derived from a single cell; pertaining to a single clone.

Monocyte. A large white blood cell with a single round nucleus. Part of the immune system.

MR or MRI (Magnetic Resonance Imaging). A diagnostic test that creates an image of body tissue by measuring the magnetic resonance of the nucleus of cells; the image is processed by mini-computer for reconstruction display.

Muscularis. The intermediate layer of the bowel wall.

Mutations. A step-by-step change in cells from a benign state to a malignant state.

Neuroblastoma. A sarcoma (a malignant condition in the connective tissues) of the nervous system, affecting mostly infants and children.

Nucleotide. The building blocks of chromosomes and DNA. A nucleotide consists of a base, a sugar, and a phosphate.

Nucleus. A spheroid body within a cell; the germ center, where the DNA exists.

Ocular melanoma. Melanoma of the eye.

Oncogene. Viral genetic material carrying the potential of cancer and passed from parent to offspring.

Oncologist. A doctor who specializes in the study of tumors.

Ovum. Female germ cell (seed) containing 46 chromosomes, which are reduced to 23 by meiosis before joining with the male sperm at fertilization.

Pancreas. An organ that secretes digestive enzymes and the hormone insulin.

Pathologist. An expert in cell structure, behavior, and cell growth. A pathologist recognizes normal and abnormal cells, such as cancer cells.

Pathology report. A report from the pathologist.

Photoelectron. An electron emitted from a metallic surface when the surface is illuminated with light; used in conjunction with the microscope, which allows for visualization of DNA.

Plastic surgery. Surgery that restores, reconstructs, corrects, or improves the shape and appearance of body structures that are defective, damaged, or misshapened by injury, disease, or growth and development.

Prednisone. A synthetic form of cortisone, a steroid that influences the nutrition and growth of connective tissues.

Primary-care physician. A doctor who specializes in family medicine and is the initial contact for care.

Prognosis. A forecast as to the probable outcome of a disease.

Protein sequenator. A method by which a gene or chromosome can be analyzed as to its composition.

Proton-beam accelerator. Equipment designed to deliver X rays at extremely high intensity and velocity.

Pulmonary embolus. A clot or other plug that obstructs the circulation to the lungs.

Radiation therapy. A cancer treatment that uses powerful doses of high-energy radiation to kill cancer cells.

Radical mastectomy. Surgery that removes the entire breast and its attachments, including the muscles of the thorax and the contents of the axilla except the main arteries and nerves. It is a disfiguring operation.

Radio sensitive. A type of cancer that responds well to X ray.

Radioactive. A substance that emits X rays.

Radiologist. A doctor who specializes in radiology. The diagnostic radiologists deal only in diagnosis; radiology oncologists treat tumors.

Receptor. A portion of cell-wall protein that responds to specific antibodies and allows entrance with toxic substances for the offending invader, be it cancer or a virus or bacteria.

Recurrence. Return of the cancer either at the original site or at a different one.

Regional recurrence. Reappearance of the cancer, usually in the lymph nodes close to the original tumor.

Rhabdomyosarcoma. A highly malignant tumor of the muscle, located in an extremity.

Shingles (herpes zoster). A virus infection that indicates a suppression of the immune system.

Sigmoid colon. Portion of the large bowel immediately above the rectum.

Sperm. Male germ cell (seed) containing 46 chromosomes, which are reduced to 23 by meiosis before joining with the female ovum at fertilization.

Spontaneous remissions. Disappearance of a disease for no explainable reason. In cancer this is rare, but it does happen.

Suture. Material used in closing a surgical or traumatic wound with stitches.

Synthesize. The artificial building of a chemical compound by the union of its elements or from other suitable starting materials.

T Cell. The most important cell in the immune system. It is the commanding general and directs the battle against the invader. It is called the floating brain.

Technology. Scientific knowledge.

Therapeutic. Curative, pertaining to the art of healing.

Tumor necrosis factor. A product that invades a cancer and causes it to disintegrate by initiating a factor resulting in death of the tumor.

Ultrasound. A diagnostic procedure that provides a visualization of deep structures of the body by recording the reflections (echoes) of pulses of ultrasonic waves directed into the tissues.

X-ray diffraction. A means by which the molecular structure of chemicals such as amino acids can be proven.

Zygote. Cell formed by the union of a male sperm and a female ovum. This cell marks the beginning of a unique human with a complete set of chromosomes and genes— 23 from the father and 23 from the mother.

SUGGESTED BIBLIOGRAPHY

Barrett, James T. *Textbook on Immunology* (St. Louis: C. V. Moseby Co., 1983).

Hood, Leroy. "Biotechnology and Medicine of the Future." *Journal of the American Medical Association* 259, no. 12 (March 12, 1988).

Kingston, Helen M. "Genetics of Cancer." *British Medical Journal* 298 (April 22, 1989).

Moore, Keith L. *The Developing Human* (Philadelphia: W. B. Saunders, 1982).

Morra, Marion and Potts, Eve. *Choices* (New York: Avon, 1987).

Overmeyer, Robert H. "Mapping Human DNA: The Clinical Promise of the Human Genome Project." *Modern Medicine* 57 (October 1989).

Rhim, John S. "Viruses, Oncogenes, and Cancer." *Cancer Detection and Prevention* (Bethesda, Maryland: National Institutes of Health, 1988), vol. 11.

Weinberg, Robert A. "The Genetic Origins of Human Cancer." *Cancer* 61 (June 10, 1987).

INDEX

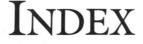

ABOUT THE AUTHOR

Born in Portland, Oregon, Dr. Paul Johnson now lives in Seattle with his wife, Genevieve. They have two grown children. He received his M.D. from Loma Linda University. He took his post-graduate training at the U.S. Public Health Service and at the Sonoma County Hospital, where he became the chief resident. He then became chief of staff and chief of surgery at Ballard Community Hospital, Seattle, Washington.

Dr. Johnson has been medical consultant for the State of Washington Department of Social and Health Services, and medical director of Personal Health of Puget Sound, an HMO. Now retired after 45 years of practicing medicine, Dr. Johnson has a weekly medical program on KIRO, Seattle's most popular radio station, and serves as public relations officer for the King County Medical Society.

Dr. Johnson is a member of the American Medical Association, the Washington State Medical Association, and the King County Medical Society. He has published three books: *Death and the Caring Community, Who Can I Turn To?* and *Spiritual Secrets to Physical Health.*